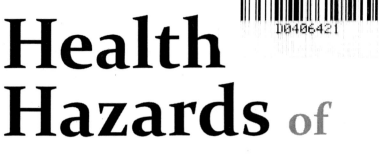

Health
Hazards of

Electromagnetic
Radiation Second Edition

A Startling Look at the Effects of Electropollution on Your Health

Edited and Compiled by
Bruce Fife, N.D.

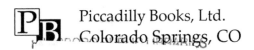

Piccadilly Books, Ltd.
Colorado Springs, CO

ACKNOWLEDGMENTS:
Much of the information in this book was compiled from data
supplied by the Electric and Magnetic Fields Research and
Public Information Dissemination Program and the National
Institute of Environmental Health Sciences.

Piccadilly Books, Ltd.
P.O. Box 25203
Colorado Springs, CO 80936, USA
www.piccadillybooks.com
orders@piccadillybooks.com

4260 0360 2/10

Library of Congress Cataloging-in-Publication Data
Fife, Bruce, 1952-
    Health hazards of electromagnetic radiation: a startling look at
the effects of electropollution on your health / Bruce Fife. -- 2nd ed.
        p. cm.
    Includes bibliographical references.
    ISBN 13: 978-0-941599-69-6
    1. Electromagnetic fields--Health aspects. 2. Electromagnetic
fields--Toxicology. I. Title.
    RA569.3.F53 2009
    363.18'9--dc22   2008037533

Printed in the USA

CONTENTS

Chapter 1

ELECTROPOLUTION

A new plague has been unleashed upon the earth—a plague that has been identified as causing various types of cancer and disrupting our body's normal biologic processes creating numerous disease-like symptoms, permanent disability, and even death. This invisible beast is so elusive that it cannot be detected by our senses, yet it is so powerful it can it can pass through solid objects—even penetrate buildings—and can travel thousands of miles at the speed of light, striking anything and everything in its path. It can be found everywhere both indoors and out. It is virtually all around us 24 hours a day. Everyone one of us are affected by it to some degree.

What is this new deadly force that has created such a ominous threat? It's electromagnetic fields (EMFs)—forces generated by the flow of electricity. With the harnessing of electrical energy and its incorporation into every aspect of our daily lives this force has become a significant threat to our health.

Electromagnetic energy surrounds and penetrate our homes, our work environment, and every place in-between. It has been accused of causing a list of effects ranging from cancer to suicide. Such a power is frightening, yet believe it or not, is totally under our control. With a flick of a switch this menacing, powerful force can be instantly knocked cold dead. Although we have the power to strike it down, we will never do it. Why? Because we have become too dependent on electricity in our everyday life. Eliminating electromagnetic fields would require the elimination of all electrical appliances and for us to go back and live like our ancestors did before the advent of electric power. This will never happen. Is there anything we can do to protect ourselves? Is it really as bad as some make it out to be? Or is it even worse that we are led to believe?

Let's face it, electricity is here to stay. If it does cause harmful effects we need to know about it and we need to know what we can do to protect ourselves. This book will try to answer these questions.

Electrical Pollution

Electricity is power. By harnessing this force we have been able to create a worldwide communications network, build machines that can perform work that would otherwise require hundreds of workers to do, and send astronauts into outer space. Electric power is a fact of life in nowadays, we have come to take for granted the simple flip of a switch that turns night into day. Electricity has made it possible to reduce manual labor, provide comfort, and entertainment, thus making life easier and more enjoyable, yet it may come with a price to pay. We all know that electric power lines, household wiring, and appliances can cause serious injury and even death from electric shock simply by touching a live wire. Researchers claim the radiation emanating from electrical appliances (e.g. electropollution) can also affect health—causing cancer, disrupt cellular function, and alter hormone levels.

A recent study from the University of North Carolina shows dangers from electromagnetic fields (EMFs) are evident in electric utility workers. The study published in the *American Journal of Epidemiology* linked elevated brain cancer rates to men who worked for long periods in exposed jobs and specifically for men who worked as linemen or electricians. Following 140,000 men at five large electric power companies in the United States form 1950 to 1986, researchers analyzed death rates in relation to magnetic field exposure history. They found brain cancer risk increased by an estimated factor of 1.94 per year of EMF exposure. The risk was 1.5 times higher for those who worked five or more years in the electrical field.

"This study is a major contribution, but it doesn't resolve the fundamental question of whether magnetic fields *cause* cancer," says David Savitz, Ph.D., study author and professor of epidemiology. Dr. Savitz is cautious about pointing to EMFs as a significant factor in cancer or other illnesses. "This study only shows an average of a two-fold increase in brain cancer. If you compare this to tobacco, which causes a twenty-fold increase in lung cancer, it doesn't appear as lethal," Savitz says.

We may wonder that if EMFs double a person's chances of getting brain cancer or some other disease isn't this enough to be worried about?

Robert O. Becker, M.D. author of *The Body Electric* and *Cross Currents* believes EMFs play a very important role in our health. "Not only is it likely that EMF effects are cancer promoting," Becker says, "but it's quite likely that chronic exposure to such fields is a competent cause for the origin of cancer."

Becker and Paul Brodeur are two of the most prominent voices in the EMF controversy. Brodeur, an investigative journalist and author of several books including *Currents of Death*, challenges the safety of power lines, VDTs (video display terminals, and home wiring. He reported that 20 percent of childhood cancers appeared traceable to exposure to a 3 mG field (previously regarded as a low, benign field).

He points out in the early 1980's in Stockholm, Sweden a survey of 2,000 homes close to power lines or substations found that the children who lived near high-current (2000,000 volt) lines had twice the incidence of cancer as those who lived farther away.

Another study in Texas showed power line workers developed brain cancer at a rate 13 times that of the general population.

Several studies in the 1980's linked unusual clusters of fetal abnormalities, birth defects and miscarriages in women with extensive video display terminal (VDT) work during pregnancy.

No one knows precisely how EMFs affect the body, let alone how they promote cancer. Many scientists remain skeptical about EMF health effects. Among them is Dimitrios Trichopoulos, chair of epidemiology at the School of Public Health. "I don't find the evidence compelling so far," he says.

Others disagree. "I think the evidence has grown stronger with time," says Dr. David Carpenter, dean of the School of Public Health at SUNY-Albany. "We have a 90 percent certainty that EMFs pose a relatively low, but significant risk of cancer," say Dr. Carpenter.

Both the U.S. government and the National Cancer Institute (NCI) are taking EMFs seriously. Recently, the NCI has contributed millions of dollars to test the hypothesis that the high breast cancer rates of industrialized nations might be explained, in part, by extensive use of electric power. And Congress has allotted $65 million for EMF research.

The question is how do electrical emissions affect our bodies? It there any effect? We all know that if you stick your finger into a light socket you will get a powerful jolt of electricity—enough to seriously burn and perhaps even kill you. But what about the electrical forces radiating out from these sources, can they also affect us physically? If so, is it harmful? These are questions scientists have been trying to answer for at least two decades. If electrical transmissions are harmful which types are the worse and how can we protect ourselves from their effects?

Electrical Radiation

A century ago scientists demonstrated that when current flows through a wire, electrical power escapes into surrounding space as waves of electromagnetic energy. This fact was used in the development of wireless transmissions and later radio and television. In fact, radio signals are also electromagnetic waves. Microwaves and X-rays are nothing more than electromagnetic energy.

In radio, television, and cellular phone transmissions electromagnetic waves are emitted by an antenna designed to focus electromagnetic forces in certain preferred directions and in certain frequency ranges. We are bombarded by these

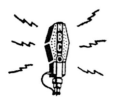 How many electrical appliances do you come in contact with each day? A major source of the electrical radiation we are exposed to comes from outside of the home or office—satellite transmissions, radio waves, power lines, etc.

electromagnetic forces constantly. However, they do not pose the greatest threat to health. The greatest threat to health for most people comes from power lines, household wiring, and electrical appliances.

Electromagnetic fields are invisible forms of energy that are created whenever electricity is flowing. Whether it is an outdoor power line, the wiring in the walls of your home, or in an appliance, like a telephone or computer, if electricity is being used, then EMFs are being generated and radiating out from the device into the surrounding environment. EMFs are able to penetrate almost all conductive materials, including metals, trees, and buildings. Even though we cannot see these waves of energy, they are very real and quite easily measured with the correct equipment.

Unlike the energy from a laser which focuses all its energy along a narrow beam, electromagnetic energy radiates out in all directions from its source. It's similar to the waves generated by a stone thrown into a quiet pool of water. Waves radiate everywhere. Electrical energy emitted from a source travels outward interacting with everything it comes into contact with, whether it be an antenna, tree, house, or human body.

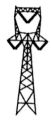

Chapter 2

ELECTRIC POWER

Electric Power Basics

In order to understand the possible threat electricity may present, it is helpful to know a little bit about what it is and how it works.

It will be helpful for you to become familiar with six basic electrical terms:

conductor

current

voltage

load

power

circuit

The *conductor* is the wire you see between power poles or

Electrical Terms	Familiar Comparisons
■ **Voltage**. Electrical pressure, the potential to do work. Measured in volts (V) or in kilovolts (kV), 1 kV = 1000 volts.	Hose connected to an open faucet but with the nozzle turned off.

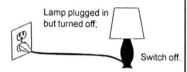

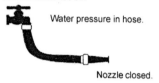

Lamp plugged in but turned off;

Switch off.

Water pressure in hose.

Nozzle closed.

■ **Current**. The movement of electric charge (e.g., electrons). Measured in amperes (A).

Hose connected to an open faucet *and* with the nozzle turned on.

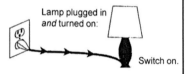

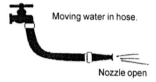

Lamp plugged in *and* turned on:

Switch on.

Moving water in hose.

Nozzle open

■ **Power.** The product of volts and current. Measured in watts (W). In the above example:

$$120 \text{ V} \times 1 \text{ A} = \textbf{120 W}$$

You can raise the voltage and lower the current and produce the same power:

$$240 \text{ V} \times 0.5 \text{ A} = \textbf{120 W}$$

Low pressure and large hose.

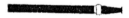

High pressure and small hose.   Same water output.

■ **Conductor.** Material that will carry electric current.

Excellent conductor: **Copper**
Fair conductor: **Human body**
Nonconductor (an insulator): **Rubber**

Good conductor: open hose.

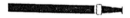

Poor conductor: kinked hose.

towers; it carries the electricity. *Current* is the movement of electrons in the conductor. *Voltage* is the electric force that causes current in a conductor.

Load is the electric power needed by homes and businesses. When a conductor energized with voltage is connected to a load, a *circuit* is completed, and *current* will flow. Electrical terms are summarized on page 12 in a comparison with more familiar examples involving water.

Electric Power Facilities

Since the strongest man-made electro-magnetic forces we encounter every day are generated by electric power plants and transmitted to our homes and places of work by power lines this source of electrical radiation has the greatest effect on our bodies.

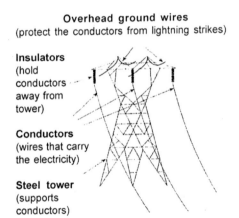

Overhead ground wires
(protect the conductors from lightning strikes)

Insulators
(hold conductors away from tower)

Conductors
(wires that carry the electricity)

Steel tower
(supports conductors)

There are two basic types of power lines: transmission lines and distribution lines. *Transmission lines* are high-voltage power lines. These are the tall metal towers we see that look much like the Eiffel tower. These towers are made more noticeable because they run along narrow strips of land free of trees and buildings, regardless of surrounding population. The utility has the right-of-way on this land so they can operate and maintain the transmission lines. These rights enable the utility to keep the right-of-way clear of trees, structures, and fire hazards that could compromise the reliability of the line and the safety of employees and the public.

The high voltage in the lines held by these towers allows electric power to be carried efficiently over long distances from electrical generation facilities to substations near urban areas. In the United States, most transmission lines use alternating current (AC) and operate at voltages between 50 and 765 kV (1kV or kilovolt=1000V).

Utilities use lower-voltage *distribution lines* to bring power from substations to businesses and homes. Distribution lines operate at voltages below 50 kV. For residential customers, these levels are further reduced to 120/240 V once the power reaches its destination.

Electrical *substations* serve many functions in controlling and transferring power on an electrical system. Several different types of equipment may be present, depending on the functions of the particular substation. For example, *transformers* change the high voltages used by transmission lines to the lower voltages used by distribution lines. *Circuit breakers* are used to turn lines on and off.

Alternating Current and Direct Current

All electrically powered appliances operate either with batteries or by plugging into the household wiring. Appliances that are powered by batteries are run by direct current (DC)—that is, the current delivered to the appliance run in only one direction. Appliances that use the power from transmission lines—the type in your home or workplace—is called alternating current (AC). The electrical current in the home is not direct

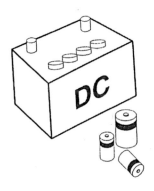 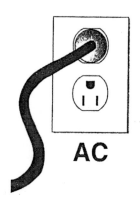

like DC but alternates one way and than the other. The current flows back and forth, but very quickly at a rate of 60 cycles each second. So although the current momentarily stops between each cycle, the interruption is so brief it has essentially no noticeable effect on the operation of electrical equipment. The reason for AC is because it can be utilized in more ways than DC can and many electrical components used in appliances rely on this type of current to operate.

Cycles per second are usually expressed in hertz or Hz, so that 60 cycles per second equals 60 Hz.

AC fields induce weak electric currents in conducting objects, including humans; DC fields do not, unless the DC field changes

---

Electric Fields

1. Produced by **voltage**.

Lamp plugged in but turned off. Voltage produces an electric field.

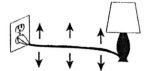

2. Measured in volts per meter (V/m) or in kilovolts per meter (kV/m).

3. **Easily shielded** (weakened) by conducting objects like trees and buildings.

4. Reduced in strength with increasing distance from the source.

---

in space or time relative to the person in the field (i.e., the person moves across the field or the strength of the field fluctuates). In most practical situations, a battery-operated appliance is unlikely to induce electric current in the person using the appliance. Induced currents from AC fields have been a focus for research on how EMFs could affect human health.

EMFs

Power lines, electrical wiring, and appliances all produce electric and magnetic fields. EMFs are invisible lines of force that surround any electrical device. Electric and magnetic fields have different properties and possibly different ways of causing biological effects. Note that while *electric* fields are easily shielded or weakened by conducting objects (e.g., trees, buildings, and

16

Magnetic Fields

1. Produced by **current**.

Lamp plugged in and turned on. Current now also produces a magnetic field.

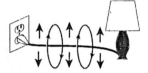

2. Measured in gauss (G).

3. **Not easily shielded** (weakened) by most material.

4. Reduced in strength with increasing distance from the source.

---

human skin), *magnetic* fields are not. However, both electric and magnetic fields weaken with increasing distance from the source.

Even though electric and magnetic fields are present around appliances and power lines, more recent interest and research have focused on potential health effects of magnetic fields. This is because epidemiological* studies have found associations between increased cancer risk and power-line configurations, which are thought to be surrogates for magnetic fields. No such associations have been found with measured electric fields.

---

* Epidemiology is a type of research which studies the patterns and possible causes of diseases in human populations. Epidemiologist study short-term epidemics such as outbreaks of food poisoning and long-term disease such as cancer and heart disease.

X-rays, about 1 billion billion Hz, can penetrate the body and damage internal organs and tissues by damaging important molecules such as DNA. This process is called "ionization."

Microwaves, at frequencies of several billion Hz, can have "thermal" or heating effects on body tissues.

Power-frequency EMF, 50 or 60 Hz, carries very little energy, has no ionizing effects and usually no thermal effects. It can, however, cause very weak electric currents to flow in the body.

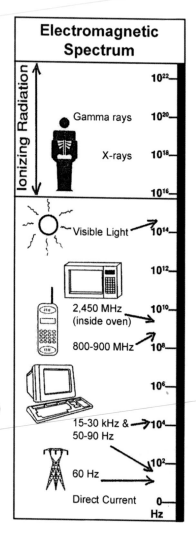

Electromagnetic Spectrum

Ionizing Radiation

Gamma rays — 10^{22}

— 10^{20}

X-rays — 10^{18}

— 10^{16}

Visible Light — 10^{14}

— 10^{12}

2,450 MHz (inside oven) — 10^{10}

800-900 MHz — 10^{8}

— 10^{6}

15-30 kHz & 50-90 Hz — 10^{4}

— 10^{2}

60 Hz

Direct Current — 0

Hz

The higher the frequency, the more rapidly the field varies. The fields do not vary at 0 Hz (direct current) and vary trillions of times per second near the top of the spectrum. Note that 104 means 10 x 10 x 10 x 10 or 10,000 Hz. 1 kilohertz (kHz) = 1,000 Hz. 1 megahertz (MHz) = 1,000,000 Hz.

Power-Frequency EMF

The electromagnetic spectrum (see page 18) covers an enormous range of frequencies. These frequencies are expressed in cycles per second (Hz). Electric power (60 Hz in North America, 50 Hz in most other places) is in the extremely-low-frequency range, which includes frequencies below 3000 Hz.

The higher the frequency, the shorter the distance between one wave and the next, and the greater the amount of energy in the field. Microwave frequency field, with wavelength of several inches, have enough energy to cause heating in conducting material. Still higher frequencies like X-rays cause ionization—the breaking of molecular bonds, which damages genetic material. In comparison, power line frequency fields have wavelengths of more than 3100 miles and consequently have very low energy levels that do not cause heating or ionization. However, AC fields do create weak electric currents in conducting objects, including people and animals.

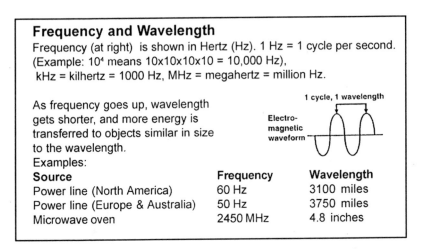

Frequency and Wavelength
Frequency (at right) is shown in Hertz (Hz). 1 Hz = 1 cycle per second. (Example: 10^4 means 10x10x10x10 = 10,000 Hz), kHz = kilhertz = 1000 Hz, MHz = megahertz = million Hz.

As frequency goes up, wavelength gets shorter, and more energy is transferred to objects similar in size to the wavelength.
Examples:

Source	Frequency	Wavelength
Power line (North America)	60 Hz	3100 miles
Power line (Europe & Australia)	50 Hz	3750 miles
Microwave oven	2450 MHz	4.8 inches

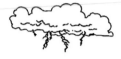

Earth's DC electric field comes from thunderstorms.

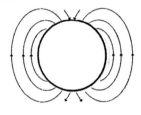

Earth's DC magnetic field comes from currents in the earth.

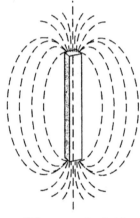

DC magnetic field around a bar magnet.

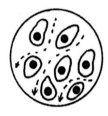

Most of the 60-Hz current occurs between the cells, not through them.

Natural EMFs

The earth produces EMFs, mainly in the form of DC (also called static fields). This is often seen in nature as static electricity. Lightening is static electricity. Electric fields are produced by thunderstorm activity in the atmosphere. Near the ground, the DC electric field averages less than 200 volts per meter (V/m). Much stronger fields, typically about 50,000 V/m, occur directly beneath electrical storms.

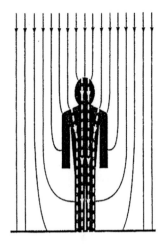 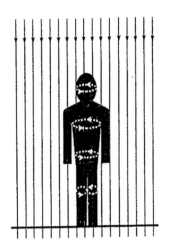

A person standing in an electric field (solid lines) showing induced current (white dashed lines).

A person standing in a magnetic field (solid lines) showing induced current (white dashed lines).

Magnetic fields are thought to be produced by electric currents flowing deep within the earth's molten core. The DC magnetic field averages around 500 milligauss (mG). This number is larger than typical AC electric power magnetic fields, but DC fields do not create currents in objects, like human bodies, in the way the AC fields do (see illustrations above).

AC fields create weak electric currents in the bodies of people and animals. This is one reason why there is a potential for EMFs to cause biological effects. As shown above, currents from electric and magnetic fields are distributed differently within the body. The amount of this current, even if you are directly beneath a large transmission line, is extremely small (millionths of an ampere). The current is too weak to penetrate cell membranes; it is present mostly between the cells.

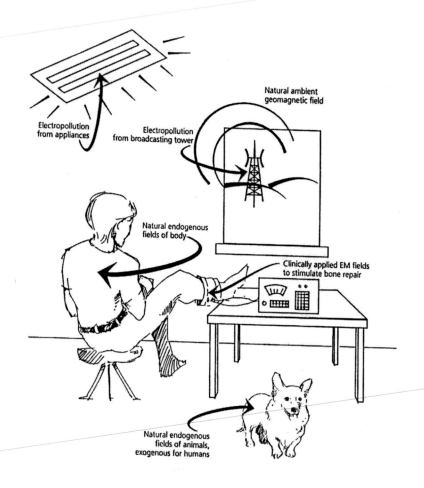

Examples of natural and created EM fields exogenous and endogenous.

Our bodies are electrical organisms. All chemical reactions within the body are electrical reactions. The body itself generates an electric field just as the earth does. This electric field can be altered by EMFs emitted from AC devices and transmission lines. As part of the normal function of our bodies, we are constantly generating extremely small electrical currents within our bodies. Our nerve impulses, which regulate all our bodily functions, are electrical signals. It is this internal electrical activity that is analyzed by medical equipment such as EEG, ECG and EMG. Principles of physics tells us that when a small electric current is in close proximity to a large EMF, the small electric current will be altered. It is believed that this alteration of our body's internal current is the reason why EMFs affect us.

Currents from 60 Hz EMFs are weaker than natural currents in the body, such as those from the electrical activity of the brain and heart. Some scientists argue that it is therefore impossible for EMFs to have any important effects on our bodies. Other scientists argue that, just as a trained ear can pick up a familiar voice or cry in a crowd, so a cell may respond to induced current as a signal, lower in intensity, yet detectable even through the background "noise" of the body's natural currents. Numerous laboratory studies have shown that biological effects can be caused by exposure to EMFs. In most cases, however, it is not clear how EMFs actually produce these demonstrated effects.

Strong electric fields, such as those found beneath large transmission lines (50-765 kV), can cause hair on your exposed head or arms to vibrate slightly at 60 Hz. This is felt by some people as a tingling sensation. EMFs from transmission lines can also, in some circumstances, cause nuisance shocks from voltages created by EMFs on objects like ungrounded metal fences.

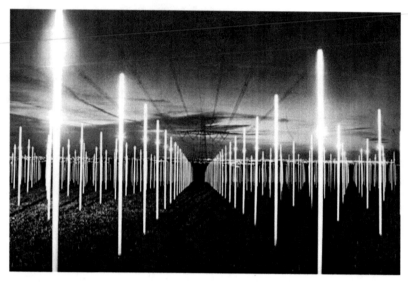

Fluorescent tubes powered by the electromagnetic field surrounding overhead power lines. Photo from RichardBox.com.

For years people have been amused by the fact that they can take a fluorescent bulb in their bare hands, go near a power line, hold it up in the air, and watch it light up. The electromagnetic field surrounding the overhead power line is strong enough light the fluorescent bulb without any additional electricity. The photo above dramatically illustrates this phenomenon. In this photo hundreds of fluorescent tubes are positioned underneath a power line and inserted into the ground by about 6 inches. The fluorescent tubes light up brightly from the energy emanating from the power line.

If you walk toward a tube positioned as shown in the photo, the light will dim and may go out. If you move away, the tube will light up again. This is because your body is a better conductor of the electromagnetic radiation than the air is, so your body shorts out this potential to the ground.

When you pass under a power line you may even feel the energy radiate through your body. Your hair may stand on end and you may hear a hum. If you touch metal it may even give you a shock. This is most likely if you walk near a power line when it is raining or damp and are holding an umbrella. The umbrella can act like an antenna of sorts, picking up the energy from the power line. You may actually hear the buzzing sound of the electricity as it flows into the umbrella. If you touch any metal on the umbrella you will get a shock. The power of the shock can be significant so I wouldn't recommend that you try it. It has been described it as a jolt similar to what you would experience by touching an electric fence. The force of the shock would vary depending on the humidity. When the humidity is high the potential for getting shocked is greater.

The danger isn't just when carrying an umbrella but when you are in contact with any metal object. Metal is an excellent conductor. Any time you pass near a power line, especially if the humidity is high, there is a potential for getting shocked. People riding motorcycles underneath power lines have reported getting shocked when they touched the aluminum hand levers with bare hands.

If the EMF from power lines is strong enough to create physical disturbances in our bodies (raising hair) and environment (electrical shocks) it seems logical to assume it can also affect the flow of electrical currents in our bodies. Therefore, electromagnetic fields have the ability to affect our health.

Chapter 3

HUMAN HEALTH STUDIES

Researchers have linked EMF exposure to ailments such as chronic fatigue syndrome, brain cancer, leukemia, breast and testicular cancer, and neurological disorders among others. Electromagnetic fields are electrical and magnetic fields that exist naturally—generated by the earth, sun, moon and even our own bodies. The activity of every living cell is our bodies is regulated by the electromagnetic field. Our metabolism is geared to natural levels of radiation and electromagnetic energies from our surroundings. The earth's electromagnetic field pulses at the rate of 7.83 Hertz (Hz), and our body's bioelectrical system pulses at about the same rate. Robert Becker, M.D. say moderate EMF exposure can produce negative biological effects, he says "[Studies] have demonstrated effects on the calcium channel permeability of cell membranes, which can affect a variety of cell functions, including the transmission of electric signals to the nerve tissue." Any deviation from normal may disrupt natural processes and therefore create cellular dysfunction and possibly disease.

Of children (ages 14 and under) in the United States, about 14 in 100,000 develop some form of cancer each year. Almost one-third of these cancers are acute lumphocytic leukemia, the most common form of leukemia in children. For childhood leukemia victims, chances of survival are about 60 percent.

Several studies have analyzed a possible association between proximity to power lines and various types of childhood cancer. Most, but not all, have reported positive associations between proximity to power lines and some forms of cancer. A few have also shown a statistically significant association with leukemia.

The first study to report an association between power lines and cancer was conducted in 1979 in Denver by Dr. Nancy Wertheimer and Ed Leeper. They found that children who had died from cancer were 2 to 3 times more likely to have lived within 131 feet of a high-current power line than were the other children studied. Exposure to magnetic fields was identified as a possible factor in this finding. Magnetic fields were not measured in the study. Instead, the researchers devised a substitute method to estimate the magnetic fields produced by the power lines. The estimate was based on the size and number of power line wires and the distance between the power lines and the home.

A second Denver study in 1988, and a 1991 study in Los Angeles, also found significant associations between living near high-current power lines and childhood cancer incidence. The L.A. study found an association with leukemia but did not look at all cancers. The 1988 Denver study found an association with all cancer incidence. When leukemia was analyzed separately, the risk was elevated but not statistically significant. In neither of these two studies were the associations found to be statistically significant when magnetic fields were measured in the home and used in the analysis.

Studies in Sweden (1992) and Mexico (1993) also found increased leukemia incidence for children living near transmission lines. A 1993 Danish study, like the 1988 Denver study, found an association for incidence of all childhood cancers but not specifically leukemia. A Finnish study found an association with central nervous system tumors in boys. Eight studies have examined risk of cancer for adults living near power lines. Of these, two found significant associations with cancer.

Swedish Studies

In late 1992, researchers in Sweden reported results of a study of cancer in people living near high-voltage transmission lines. The Swedish study generated a great deal of interest among scientists, the public, and the news media. Relative risk for leukemia increased in Swedish children who lived within 164 feet of a transmission line. The risk was found also to increase progressively as the calculated average annual 50 Hz magnetic field increased in strength. However, the risk calculations were based on a very small number of cases.

The Swedish researchers concluded that their study provides additional evidence for a possible link between magnetic fields and childhood leukemia. However, scientists have expressed differing opinions about this study. Some scientists believe the study is important because it is based on magnetic field levels presumed to have existed around the time the cancers were diagnosed. Others are skeptical because of the small numbers

Summary of Swedish Residential Cancer Study

- Cancer cases (from 1960-85) and controls were selected from the 500,000 people who had lived on property within 984 ft of 220- and 400 kV lines.
- Magnetic field exposure was estimated by (1) in-home measurements, (2) dwelling distance from lines, and (3) calculated average annual magnetic field before and near time of cancer diagnosis.
- The trend for increasing risk of child leukemia with increasing field strength was statistically significant.
- No cancer association was found with present-day in-home magnetic field measurements.
- For homes within 164 feet of transmission lines, relative risk for childhood leukemia was borderline significant.
- Excess leukemia risks were found only in one-family homes. There were no elevated risks for other types of child cancers.
- Control for possible effects of air pollution and socioeconomic status did not change study results.
- Adults with highest cumulative exposures to power line EMFs had twice the risk of developing acute or chronic myeloid leukemia.

Source: Feychting & Ahlbom 1992, 1993

of cancer cases and because no cancer association was seen with present-day magnetic field levels measured in the home.

The National Electrical Safety Board of Sweden estimates that if, as this study suggest, living near overhead transmission lines increases a child's risk of developing leukemia, then approximately two children per year in Sweden would develop leukemia as a result of living near such power lines. There are about 70 new cases of childhood leukemia per year in Sweden.

Information on adult cancer incidence was also collected and analyzed in the Swedish study. Researchers reported in 1994 that adults with the highest cumulative exposure (over 15 years) to power-line EMFs were twice as likely to develop acute or chronic myeloid leukemia as were less exposed adults. Although the total number of cases were small, which made the results of borderline statistical significance, the study provides some evidence for an association between exposure to magnetic fields from power lines and acute and chronic myeloid leukemia in adults.

Cluster Cases

Scientists call unusual occurrences of cancer in an area or in time a "cancer cluster." In some cases, a cancer cluster has served as an early warning of a health hazard. For most reports of cancer clusters, however, the cause is never determined, or the perceived cluster is not really an unusual occurrence.

As an analogy, think about how an uncommon family name might be distributed at homes located throughout a city. Would it be unusual to find neighborhoods where two or three unrelated families with this same name live in the same small area? Statistically, this may be shown to be expected due just to chance. While four or more such families may be very unlikely due to chance, this does not mean that it is impossible. One possible cause (other than chance) for some such "name clusters" is that the families are part of the same ethnic group, and they choose to live close together. For perceived neighborhood cancer clusters, however, health agencies generally never find a common environmental cause. It is also apparent that the definition of a "cluster" depends on how large an area (neighborhood) is included.

Concerns have been raised about seemingly high numbers of cancers in some neighborhoods and schools close to electric power facilities. In recent years, three state health departments have studied apparent cancer clusters near electric power facilities. A Connecticut study involved five cases of brain and

Cancer cases (x's on diagram) in a city may show patterns that appear to be "clusters." They may seem to suggest a common environmental cause. Usually such patterns are due just to chance. Further, delineation of a cluster is subjective—where do you draw the circles?

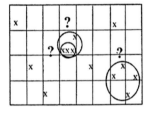

central nervous system cancers in people living near an electrical substation. The local rates for these types of cancer were found to be no different from statewide rates. Examination of cancer rates at various distances for the substation also failed to show evidence of clustering. In North Carolina, several cases of brain cancer were identified in part of a county that included an electric power generating plant. An investigation showed that brain cancer rates in the county, however, were actually lower than statewide rates. Among staff at an elementary school near transmission lines in California, 13 cancers of various types

31

were identified. Although this was twice the expected rate, the state investigators concluded that it was possible that the cancers could have occurred by chance alone.

Electrical Workers

Several studies have reported increased cancer risks for jobs involving work around electrical equipment. To date, it is not clear whether these risks are caused by EMFs or by other factors. A report published in 1982 by Dr. Samuel Milham was one of the first to suggest that electrical workers have a higher risk of leukemia than do workers in other occupations. The Milham study was based on death certificates from Washington state and included workers in 10 occupations assumed to have elevated exposure to EMFs. A subsequent study by Milham, published in 1990, reported elevated levels of leukemia and lymphoma among workers in aluminum smelters, which use very large amounts of electrical power.

The effects of EMF on cancer are still being debated. About 50 studies have now reported statistically significant increased risks for several types of cancer in occupational groups presumed to have elevated exposure to EMFs. Relative risk levels in these studies are mostly small, and the possible influence of other factors such as chemicals has not been ruled out. At least 30 other studies did *not* find any significant cancer risks in electrical workers. Most of the earlier occupational studies did not include actual measurements of EMF exposure on the job. Instead, they used, "electrical" job titles as indicators of assumed elevated exposure to EMFs. Recent studies, however, have included extensive EMF exposure assessments.

A report published in 1992 by Dr. Joseph Bowman and colleagues provided some information about actual EMF exposures of various electrical workers. As shown in the table below, electrical workers in Los Angeles and Seattle did have higher EMF exposures than nonelectrical workers.

EMF Exposures of Workers in Los Angeles and Seattle				
Job Type	Mean Electric Field		Mean Magnetic Field	
	Los Angeles	Seattle	Los Angeles	Seattle
Elcetrical	19.0 V/m	51.2 V/m	9.6 mG	27.6 mG
Nonelectrical	5.5 V/m	10.6 V/m	1.7 mG	4.1 mG

There are two common ways of describing a middle value in a sample of measurements: **Mean** = The sum of all measurements in a sample divided by the number of measurements. **Median** = The middle measurement in a sample arranged in order of size. There are as many measurements larger than the median as there are smaller. The median is useful for data with some very high or very low measurements.

For this study, the category "electrical workers" included electrical engineering technicians, electrical engineers, electricians, power line and cable workers, power station operators, telephone line workers, TV and radio repairmen, and welders and flame cutters.

In a further analysis published in July 1994, Dr. Stephanie London, Bowman, and others found a weakly positive trend for increased leukemia risk in relation to exposure to magnetic fields among electrical workers in Los Angeles County. These results were consistent with findings from studies based on job title alone that electrical workers may be at slightly increased risk of leukemia.

A 1993 study (Sahl, et al.) of 36,000 electrical workers at a large utility in California found no consistent evidence of an association between measured magnetic fields and cancer. Some elevated risks for lymphoma and leukemia were observed, but they were not statistically significant. A 1992 study of Swedish workers (Floderus, et al.) found an association between average EMF exposure and chronic lymphocytic leukemia but not acute myeloid leukemia. There was some evidence of increasing risk with increasing exposure. The Floderus study also reported an increase in brain tumors among younger men whose work involved relatively high magnetic field exposure.

Results of major study of electrical workers in Canada and France were reported in early 1994. The research team, led by Dr. Gilles Theriault, looked at 4151 cancer cases in 233,292 workers from two utilities in Canada and one in France. Workers with more than the median cumulative magnetic field exposure (31 mG) had a significantly higher (up to three times higher) risk of developing acute myeloid leukemia. Workers who had the greatest exposures to magnetic fields had twelve times the expected rate of astrocytomas (a type of brain tumor), but according to the authors, this finding "suffered from serious statistical limits" and was based on a small number of cases (five) in the highest exposure category. In the analysis of median cumulative magnetic field exposure, no significant elevated risks were found for the other 29 types of cancer studied.*

There were inconsistencies in results among the three utilities and no clear indication of a dose-response trend. The authors concluded, therefore, that their results did not provide definitive evidence that magnetic fields were the cause of the elevated risks found in leukemia and brain cancer. However, they

---

* A later analysis reported an association between exposure to short bursts of extremely high magnetic fields and increased risk of lung cancer.

observed as "noteworthy" the fact that despite the enormous number of analyses done, the only two types of cancer for which a significant association with EMF was found (leukemia and brain cancer) were among the three for which an association had been hypothesized, based on previous studies.

In another major study involving more than 138 utility workers (Savitz, et al. 1995), the authors concluded that the results "do not support an association between occupational magnetic field exposure and leukemia, but do suggest a link to brain cancer."

Breast Cancer

There is some epidemiological evidence for an association between EMF exposure and breast cancer, but studies have also reported evidence to the contrary.

A 1994 study (Loomis et al.) examined death records of female workers and found that women employed in electrical occupations were slightly more likely to have died of breast cancer than were other working women. However, because the study could not control for factors such as diet, fertility, and family history (which are known to affect breast cancer risk), the results are considered to be preliminary, not conclusive. A 1994 Norwegian study reported an excess risk of breast cancer among female radio and telegraph operators abroad ships. A 1993 Danish study found no association between occupational EMF exposure and female breast cancer. Several studies have reported an increased risk of breast cancer among men employed in EMF-related occupations. However, the 1994 study of electrical workers in Canada and France reported no such association.

Other Health Problems

Several epidemiologic studies have looked for EMF effects on pregnancy outcomes and general health. Various EMF sources have been studied for possible association with miscarriage risk: power lines and substations, electric blankets, and heated water beds, electric cable ceiling heat, and computer monitors or video display terminals (VDTs). Some studies have correlated EMF exposure with higher than expected miscarriage rates; others have found no such correlation. Epidemiologic studies have revealed no evidence of an association between EMF exposure and birth defects in humans.

Several studies looked at the overall health of high-voltage electrical workers, and a few looked at the incidence of suicide or depression in people living near transmission lines. Results

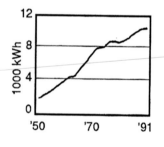

U.S. per capita electricity sales from 1950 to 1991 (Kujawa, et al. 1992)

of these studies have been mixed. Some studies have also investigated the possibility that certain sensitive individuals may experience allergic-type reactions to EMFs, known as "electrosensitivity."

One report released in 1994 has suggested a possible link between occupational EMF exposure and increased incidence of Alzheimer's disease among tailors and dressmakers.

Laboratory Studies

Several kinds of biological effects have been reported in studies of electric and/or magnetic fields. A biological effect is a measurable change in some biological factor. It may or may not have any bearing on health. Overall, effects attributed to EMFs have been small and difficult to reproduce. Very specific laboratory conditions are usually needed for effects of EMFs to be detected. It is not known how EMFs actually cause these effects.

Laboratory studies to date have not answered questions about possible human health effects. These studies are, however, providing clues about how EMFs interact with basic biological processes. The cell membrane may be an important site of interaction with induced currents from EMFs.

Keep in mind that some of these effects are within the "normal" range of variation. A biological response to a particular stimulus does not necessarily result in a negative health effect.

Melatonin is a hormone produced mainly at night by the pineal, a small gland in the brain. One reason scientists are interested in melatonin is that it could help explain results of some EMF epidemiological studies. Melatonin has been reported to slow the growth of some cancer cells, including breast cancer cells, in laboratory experiments. If power-frequency EMF can affect melatonin in humans, this could be a mechanism to explain results of some EMF studies of breast cancer.

Effects of 60 Hz EMFs Reported in Some Laboratory Studies
• Changes in functions of cells and tissues • Decrease in the hormone melatonin • Alternations of immune system • Accelerated tumor growth • Changes in biorhythms • Changes in human brain activity and heart rate

Laboratory studies have shown that it is unlikely that EMFs can *initiate* the cancer process. Some studies suggest, however, that power-frequency EMFs may *promote* development of certain existing cancers.

In the 1980s, scientists found that in rats exposed to 60 Hz electric fields, nighttime melatonin levels were reduced. Other studies have since reported that both AC and DC magnetic fields can also affect melatonin levels in rats and hamsters. These experiments are very delicate and depend on a combination of factors such as age of the animals and length of day. Melatonin levels were not affected in sheep raised for nearly a year in the EMFs directly beneath a 500 kV transmission line. Experiments with baboons also showed no changes in melatonin. The Midwest Research Institute (MRI) has studied the effect of 60 Hz magnetic field exposure on human melatonin. In 1993 MRI reported that although subjects showed no effect on the average, those individuals with naturally lower levels of melatonin did show a small further decrease. However, in 1994 MRI reported that a second study, specifically designed to replicate the earlier results, found no such effect.

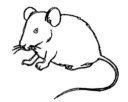

Melatonin

What Is Melatonin?

The daily secretion of the hormone melatonin by the pineal gland is driven by a natural generator in the brain. Light regulates the generator so the melatonin secretion by the pineal matches the day-night cycle. Melatonin levels are very low during the day and increase rapidly at night. The secretion corresponds to the length of the day and night. This provides biological information about the time of day and time of year.

What Does It Do?

Regulation of Seasonal Breeding

Wildlife and many domestic species such as sheep breed only at certain times of the year. Melatonin provides the animals' reproductive system with the necessary time-of-year information. If melatonin patterns are altered, the timing of reproduction can be affected.

Regulation of Circadian Rhythms

Melatonin helps regulate daily biological rhythms such as the sleep-wake cycle. It also appears to influence mood and behavior. Some types of depression and "jet lag" may be related to irregularities in the melatonin rhythm.

Tumor Suppression

Melatonin seems to have an antitumor effect. In some studies, breast cancer in women was associated with low levels of melatonin. Some animal and cell studies also found that melatonin helps reduce the growth of tumors.

What Affects It?

Under certain conditions, nighttime melatonin can be depressed by lack of daytime sunlight, stress, alcohol, and EMF.

Laboratory Animals

Studies found that 60 Hz magnetic fields reduced melatonin levels in test animals. Exposure to the field as brief as only 15 minutes was all that was needed to create a measurable difference.

Sheep

A study on sheep found no effects of EMF on melatonin in sheep raised beneath a transmission line. However, a possible effect on the immune system was found.

Humans

One study suggested melatonin was affected in certain women using electric blankets.

Besides the possibility of causing or aggravating certain preexisting diseases such as cancer, symptoms ascribed to EMF exposure include:

- sleeplessness

- nervousness

- headaches

- allergies

- fatigue

- depression

Researcher and author Robert Becker claims that EMF exposure can:

- Increase cancer-cell division rate.

- Increase incidence of certain cancers.

- Create developmental abnormalities in embryos.

- Alter neurochemicals resulting in behavioral abnormalities such as suicide.

- Alter biological cycles.

- Encourage stress responses in exposed animals that, if prolonged, lead to declines in immune system efficiency.

- Alter learning ability.

What Does All This Mean?

After a review all of the most recent studies most scientists worldwide have concluded that the existing evidence, although suggestive, does not show *conclusive* proof that EMFs *cause* cancer. It appears that in at least some types of diseases, while EMF exposure may not necessarily *cause* a condition, it can aggravate it and make it more severe. Certain types of cancer, for example, may have been caused by other factors, but EMFs can accelerate the rate of growth. Biological testing has clearly demonstrated that EMFs *do* have an influence on cells and

---

Biological Effects of EMFs

From a report by the American Medical Association on EMFs, in laboratory tests of EMFs, using both whole animals and cell culture data, changes were present in the following measured parameters:

- The nervous system
- Ion movement across cell membranes
- Cellular enzymes
- Chromatid and chromosome structure
- Brain electrophysiology
- Perception
- Behavior: Social and operant
- Lymphocyte cytotoxicity
- Pineal gland melatonin suppression
- Circadian Rhythm (biological clock)
- Bone healing delays
- Testosterone concentration
- Brain seizure induction
- Tumor cell plating efficiency
- Brain neurotransmitter concentration
- DNA production
- Oncogene promotion
- Evoked response
- Heart rate

Source: Report 7 of the Council on Scientific Affairs, January 1994, "Effects of Electric and Magnetic Fields"

tissues. The consequences of these effects are still being debated.

The Swedish government has issued a public information document that states, "We suspect that magnetic fields may pose certain risks to health, but we cannot be certain." While research is under way to pin this down, the report continues, "there is good reason to exercise a certain amount of caution." The Swedish government recommends against locating new homes and schools near existing electricity generating plants and proposes that high magnetic fields in homes, schools, and workplaces be limited. It specifically states, however, that "current knowledge is not sufficient for us to tell how magnetic fields affect us. So we do not have a basis on which to set [exposure] limits."

A summary of all studies of both human epidemiological and biological laboratory testing has shown both adverse and benign effects associated with EMFs. Because of the conflicting results in many studies there has been a no clear cut cause and effect relationship established between certain diseases or dysfunction and EMF exposure. However, in human studies there does seem to be, at least statistically, evidence that EMF can affect health.

At this point it can be concluded that *moderate* exposure to EMFs pose a minor health hazard for most of us, but overexposure such as experienced in certain occupations or living conditions (near power lines) may contribute to a number of biological changes that could definitely affect health and help to promote disease. Besides those who are exposed to high levels of electromagnetic radiation, other groups of people who are at high risk are the very old, the very young (including unborn children), and those who suffer from chronic health conditions. Since EMFs can adversely affect these people, it must have some influence on the all of us. It would be wise to limit exposure as much as possible.

EMF Standards

In the United States, there are no federal health standards specifically for 60 Hz EMFs. At least six states have set standards for transmission line electric fields; two of these also have standards for magnetic fields. The two state magnetic field standards (New York and Florida) are basically the maximum fields that existing lines in those states produce under maximum load-carrying conditions. In other words, their purpose is to ensure that future power lines do not exceed current EMF levels.

Two organizations have developed guidelines for 60 Hz EMF exposure, as shown in the following tables. Both sets of

International Guidelines on Non-Ionizing Radiation Protection		
Exposure (50/60 Hz)	Electric Field	Magnetic Field
Occupational: Whole working day Short term[a] For limbs **General Public:** Up to 24 hours per day Few hours per day	10 kV/m 30 kV/m — 5 kV/m 10 kV/m	5 G (5,000 mG) 50 G (50,000 mG) 250 G (250,000 mG) 1 G (1,000 mG) 10 G (10,000 mG)
[a]For electric fields of 10-30 kV/m, field strength (kV/m) x hours of exposure should not exceed 80 for the whole working day. Whole-body exposure to magnetic fields up to 2 hours per day should not exceed 50 mG. Source: IRPA/INIRC 1990::		

ACGIH Occupational Threshold Limit Values for 60 Hz EMF
Electric Field Occupational exposures should not exceed: 25 kV/m (from 0 Hz to 100 Hz). Prudence dictates the use of protective devices (e. g. suits, gloves, insulation) in fields above 15 kV/m.
Magnetic Field Occupational exposure 10 G (10,000 mG) For workers with cardiac pacemakers, the field should not exceed: 1 G (1,000 mG).
Source: American Conference of Governmental Industrial Hygienists (ACGIH) 1994

guidelines are based on established effects of EMFs, such as nerve stimulation, and are much higher than EMF levels found typically in occupational and residential environments. They are not meant to correspond to the low-level field strengths associated with elevated cancer incidence reported in recent epidemiological studies and should not be interpreted as distinguishing "safe" from "unsafe" EMF levels. Researchers and regulators do not know at this point the degree to which EMF exposure from power frequency sources constitute a health hazard. Therefore, they have not yet determined levels of exposure which could be considered safe or unsafe.

Chapter 4

EMF EXPOSURE AT HOME AND AT WORK

Magnetic fields close to electrical appliances are often stronger than the fields directly beneath power lines! For example, the strength of the magnetic field directly under a power line is typically well below 100 mG, while household and office appliances can have magnetic fields many times this amount. So depending upon the type of electrical equipment you use in your home or office you could be exposed to much more electromagnetic energy than if you lived next to a power line. Fortunately however, appliance fields decrease in strength with distance more quickly than do power line fields (see graph at top of next page).

Typical EMF levels for transmission lines are shown in the chart on the bottom of the next page. At a distance of about 300 feet, at times of average electricity demand, the magnetic field from many lines can be similar to typical background EMF levels found in most homes (less than about 2 mG). As the

45

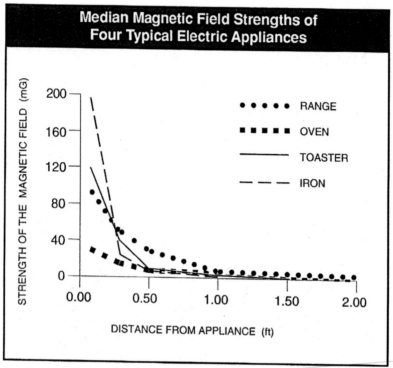

Median Magnetic Field Strengths of Four Typical Electric Appliances

STRENGTH OF THE MAGNETIC FIELD (mG)

• • • • • RANGE
■ ■ ■ ■ ■ OVEN
———— TOASTER
— — — IRON

DISTANCE FROM APPLIANCE (ft)

Strength of the magnetic field declines quickly with distance from the appliance.

chart shows, the distance at which the magnetic field from the line becomes indistinguishable from typical background EMFs differs for different types of lines. Neighborhood distribution lines can also sometimes produce significant magnetic fields, depending on the amount of current they carry.

Do you live near a electric power substation? Actually, they are not believed to be a major source of excessive EMFs. The strongest EMFs around the outside of a electric power substation come from the power lines entering and leaving the station. The strength of the EMFs from transformers decreases rapidly with increasing distance. Beyond the substation fence, the EMFs produced by the equipment within the station are typically indistinguishable from background levels.

EMF Exposures in Common Environments
Magnetic fields measured in milligauss (mG)

Environment	Median* exposure	Top 5th percentile
OFFICE BUILDING		
Support staff	0.6	3.7
Professional	0.5	2.6
Maintenance	0.6	3.8
Visitor	0.6	2.1
SCHOOL		
Teacher	0.6	3.3
Student	0.5	2.9
Custodian	1.0	4.9
Administrative staff	1.3	6.9
HOSPITAL		
Patient	0.6	3.6
Medical staff	0.8	5.6
Visitor	0.6	2.4
Maintenance	0.6	5.9
MACHINE SHOP		
Machinist	0.4	6.0
Welder	1.1	24.6
Engineer	1.0	5.1
Assembler	0.5	6.4
Office staff	0.7	4.7
GROCERY STORE		
Cashier	2.7	11.9
Butcher	2.4	12.8
Office staff	2.1	7.1
Customer	1.1	7.7

Magnetic field exposures can vary greatly from site to site for any type of environment. The data shown in this table are median measurements taken at four different sites for each environment category.

*The median of four measurements. For this table, the median is the average of the two middle measurements.

Source: National Institute for Occupational Safety and Health.

Background Magnetic Field

A typical American home has a background magnetic field level (away from any appliances) that ranges form 0.5 mG to 4 mG, with an average value of 0.9 mG. Most ordinary electrical appliances produce higher localized magnetic fields.

Several EMF epidemiological studies have used 2 or 3 mG as a cut-off point to define broad categories of exposure. Below this level, subjects are considered "unexposed," and above this level they are considered "exposed." In some studies, a higher cancer risk was found within the exposed group. Other studies found no such increased risk. The significance of 2 mG used in some studies is as a boundary to define the exposed group, not as a safety threshold. Although some experiments with cells have reported effects at field levels as low as 2 mG, there is no *laboratory evidence* for adverse human health effects below this level. This doesn't necessarily mean that 2 mG is safe. It

TRANSPORTATION		
Mode of Transport	EMF(mG)	Comments
Cars, minivans, and trucks	0.1–125	Steel-belted tires are the principal EMF source for gas/diesel vehicles.
Bus (diesel powered)	0.5–146	
Electric cars	0.1–81	
Chargers for electric cars	4–63	Measured 2 ft from charger.
Electric buses	0.1–88	Measured at waist. Fields at ankles 2-5 times higher.
Electric train passenger cars	0.1–330	Measured at waist. Fields at ankles 2-5 times higher.
Airliner	0.8–24.2	Measured at waist.

Average field (mG)	Population exposed (%) Home	Bed	Work	School	Travel
> 0.5	69	48	81	63	87
> 1	38	30	49	25	48
> 2	14	14	20	3.5	13
> 3	7.8	7.2	13	1.6	4.1
> 4	4.7	4.7	8.0	< 1	1.5
> 5	3.5	3.7	4.6		1.0
> 7.5	1.2	1.6	2.5		0.5
> 10	0.9	0.8	1.3		< 0.2
> 15	0.1	0.1	0.9		

Estimated Average Magnetic Field Exposure of the U.S. Population for Various Activities

This table shows average magnetic fields experienced during different types of activities. In general, magnetic fields are greater at work than at home.

only indicates that it appears to be relatively safe, but long term exposure may have some effect not yet determined.

The Swedish study suggested a dose/response relationship for EMF exposure: The higher the estimated magnetic field exposure, the higher the cancer risk. To deduce from the Swedish study, however, that 2 mG is some sort of safety threshold is to read far too much into the data. The Swedish government has so far concluded that current knowledge does not provide sufficient basis for setting exposure limits.

As a source of comparison with the magnetic field throughout your home, see the graph above.

This chart summarizes data from a study by the Electric Power Research Institute (EPRI) in which spot measurements

Typical EMF Levels for Transmission Lines

115 kV

	(at tower)	Approx. Edge of Right-of-way 15 m (50 ft)	30 m (100 ft)	61 m (200 ft)	91 m (300 ft)
Electric Field (kV/m)	1.0	0.5	0.07	0.01	0.003
Mean Mag. Field (mG)	29.7	6.5	1.7	0.4	0.2

230 kV

	(at tower)	Approx. Edge of Right-of-way 15 m (50 ft)	30 m (100 ft)	61 m (200 ft)	91 m (300 ft)
Electric Field (kV/m)	2.0	1.5	0.3	0.05	0.01
Mean Mag. Field (mG)	57.5	19.5	7.1	1.8	0.8

500 kV

	(at tower)	Approx. Edge of Right-of-way 20 m (65 ft)	30 m (100 ft)	61 m (200 ft)	91 m (300 ft)
Electric Field (kV/m)	7.0	3.0	1.0	0.3	0.1
Mean Mag. Field (mG)	86.7	29.4	12.6	3.2	1.4

Left: Electric fields from power lines are relatively stable because line voltage doesn't change very much. Magnetic fields on most lines fluctuate greatly as current changes in response to changing loads. Magnetic fields must be described statistically in terms of averages, maximums, etc. The magnetic fields shown are means calculated for 321 power lines. During peak loads (about 1% of the time), magnetic fields are about twice as strong as the mean levels shown.

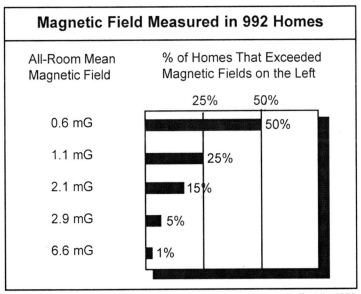

Magnetic Field Measured in 992 Homes

All-Room Mean Magnetic Field	% of Homes That Exceeded Magnetic Fields on the Left
0.6 mG	50%
1.1 mG	25%
2.1 mG	15%
2.9 mG	5%
6.6 mG	1%

Source: Zaffanella 1993

Above: The EPRI study of 992 homes was not designed to measure people's actual exposure to magnetic fields. Instead, it focused on identifying internal and external sources of these fields in the home. Your exposure to magnetic fields depends on how much time you spend near various sources and on the strength of the fields produced by those sources.

of magnetic fields were made in the center of rooms in 992 homes throughout the United States. Half of the homes studied had magnetic field measurements of 0.6 mG or less, when the average of measurements from all the rooms in the house were calculated (i.e., the all-room mean magnetic filed). The all-room mean magnetic filed for all homes studied was 0.9 mG. Only 15 percent of the homes had means magnetic fields greater than 2.1 mG. The measurements were made away from electrical appliances and primarily reflect the fields from outside power lines, household wiring, and electrical grounding sources.

Many of the childhood studies on EMFs found an association between average magnetic field levels of 2 to 3 mG and increased cancer risk. "Below that level, there is no reason for concern," says Dr. David Savitz of the University of North Carolina, who headed one of the childhood studies.

Many home appliances, for instance, emit extremely high levels of EMFs—often over 100 mG—when you are up close to them; but the field often falls off over a relatively short distance, usually within a few feet.

Household Appliances

The following tables show typical 60 Hz magnetic fields for a number of electrical appliances commonly found in homes and workplaces. Many people are surprised when they compare magnetic field measurement data from appliance to appliance and see that magnetic field strength does not depend on how large, complex, powerful, or noisy the appliance is. In fact, the magnetic fields near large appliances are often weaker than those near smaller devices. There are many reasons why this can happen, all of them related to product function and design.

In the following tables, all magnetic field measurements are given in units of milligauss (mG), and dashes in columns mean that the magnetic field measurement at this distance from the operating appliance could not be distinguished from background measurements taken before the appliance was turned on.

Kitchen Sources

Distance from Source	6"	1'	2'	4'
GARBAGE DISPOSAL				
Lowest	60	8	1	-
Median	80	10	2	-
Highest	100	20	3	-
MICROWAVE OVENS				
Lowest	100	1	1	-
Median	200	4	10	2
Highest	300	200	30	20
MIXERS				
Lowest	30	5	-	-
Median	100	10	1	-
Highest	600	100	10	-
ELECTRIC OVENS				
Lowest	4	1	-	-
Median	9	4	-	-
Highest	20	5	1	-
ELECTRIC RANGES				
Lowest	20	-	-	-
Median	30	8	2	-
Highest	200	30	9	6
REFRIGERATORS				
Lowest	-	-	-	-
Median	2	2	1	-
Highest	40	20	10	10
TOASTERS				
Lowest	5	-	-	-
Median	10	3	-	-
Highest	20	7	-	-

continued on following page

Kitchen Sources				
Distance from Source	**6"**	**1'**	**2'**	**4'**
BLENDERS				
Lowest	30	5	-	.
Median	70	10	2	.
Highest	100	20	3	.
CAN OPENERS				
Lowest	500	40	3	-
Median	600	150	20	2
Highest	1500	300	30	4
COFFEE MAKERS				
Lowest	4	-	-	-
Median	7	-	-	-
Highest	10	1	-	-
CROCK POTS				
Lowest	3	-	-	-
Median	6	1	-	-
Highest	9	1	-	-
DISHWASHERS				
Lowest	10	6	2	-
Median	20	10	4	-
Highest	100	30	7	1
FOOD PROCESSORS				
Lowest	20	5	-	-
Median	30	6	2	-
Highest	130	20	3	-

Magnetic field measurements in units of milligauss (mG).
Source: *EMF In Your Environment, EPA 1992*

Living/Family Room Sources

Distance from Source	6"	1'	2'	4'
CEILING FANS				
Lowest		-	-	-
Median		3	-	-
Highest		50	6	1
WINDOW AIR CONDITIONERS				
Lowest		-	-	-
Median		3	1	-
Highest		20	6	4
TUNERS/TAPE PLAYERS				
Lowest	-	-	-	-
Median	1	-	-	-
Highest	3	1	-	-
COLOR TVs				
Lowest		-	-	-
Median		7	2	-
Highest		20	8	4
BLACK AND WHITE TVs				
Lowest		1	-	-
Median		3	-	-
Highest		10	2	1

Magnetic field measurements in units of milligauss (mG).

Source: *EMF In Your Environment*, EPA 1992.

Laundry/Utility Room Sources				
Distance from Source	6"	1'	2'	4'
ELECTRIC CLOTHES DRYERS				
Lowest	2	-	-	-
Median	3	2	-	-
Highest	10	3	-	-
WASHING MACHINES				
Lowest	4	1	-	-
Median	20	7	1	-
Highest	100	30	6	-
IRONS				
Lowest	6	1	-	-
Median	8	1	-	-
Highest	20	3	-	-
PORTABLE HEATERS				
Lowest	5	1	-	-
Median	100	20	4	-
Highest	150	40	8	1
VACUUM CLEANERS				
Lowest	100	20	4	-
Median	300	60	10	1
Highest	700	200	50	10

Magnetic field measurements in units of milligauss (mG).
Source: *EMF In Your Environment*, EPA 1992.

Sewing machines: Home sewing machines can produce magnetic fields of 12 mG at chest level and 5 mG at head level. Magnetic fields as high as 35 mG at chest level and 215 mG at knee level have been measured from industrial sewing machines modes.

56

Bedroom Sources				
Distance from Source	6"	1'	2'	4'
DIGITAL CLOCKS				
Lowest		-	-	-
Median		1	-	-
Highest		8	2	1
ANALOG (CONVENTIONAL DIAL-FACE) CLOCKS				
Lowest		1	-	-
Median		15	2	-
Highest		30	5	3
BABY MONITORS				
Lowest	4	-	-	-
Median	6	1	-	-
Highest	15	2	-	-

Magnetic field measurements in units of milligauss (mG).
Source: *EMF In Your Environment*, EPA 1992.

Most digital clocks have low magnetic fields. In some analog clocks, however, higher magnetic fields are produced by the motor that drives the hands.

In the table, the clocks are electrically powered using AC, as are all the appliances described in these tables. The measurements for baby monitors were taken for the unit nearest the child.

Workshop Sources				
Distance from Source	**6'**	**1'**	**2'**	**4'**
BATTERY CHARGERS				
Lowest	3	2	-	-
Median	30	3	-	-
Highest	50	4	-	-
DRILLS				
Lowest	100	20	3	-
Median	150	30	4	-
Highest	200	40	6	-
POWER SAWS				
Lowest	50	9	1	-
Median	200	40	5	-
Highest	1000	300	40	4
ELECTRIC SCREWDRIVERS (while charging)				
Lowest	-	-	-	-
Median	-	-	-	-
Highest	-	-	-	-

The United States has set no standards for magnetic fields from video display terminals (VDTs)/computer monitors. The Swedish government issued guidelines recommending that VDTs purchased by the government produce magnetic fields of no more than 2.5 mG at a distance of 50 cm (approximately 1 ft, 8 in.) from the VDT surface. This Swedish government procurement standard has become a de facto standard in the VDT industry worldwide. The newer flat-screen monitors/TVs emit much less radiation.

Office Sources				
Distance from Source	**6"**	**1'**	**2'**	**4'**
AIR CLEANERS				
Lowest	110	20	3	-
Median	180	35	5	1
Highest	250	50	8	2
COPY MACHINES				
Lowest	4	2	1	-
Median	90	20	7	1
Highest	200	40	13	4
FAX MACHINES				
Lowest	4	-	-	-
Median	6	-	-	-
Highest	9	2	-	-
FLUORESCENT LIGHTS				
Lowest	20	-	-	-
Median	40	6	2	-
Highest	100	30	8	4
ELECTRIC PENCIL SHARPENERS				
Lowest	20	8	5	-
Median	200	70	20	2
Highest	300	90	30	30
VIDEO DISPLAY TERMINALS (PCs WITH COLOR MONITORS) (See note at left)				
Lowest	7	2	1	-
Median	14	5	2	-
Highest	20	6	3	-

Magnetic field measurements in units of milligauss (mG).

Source: *EMF In Your Environment*, EPA 1992.

Bathroom Sources				
Distance from Source	6"	1'	2'	4'
HAIR DRYERS				
Lowest	1	-	-	-
Median	300	1	-	-
Highest	700	70	10	1
ELECTRIC SHAVERS				
Lowest	4	-	-	-
Median	100	20	-	-
Highest	600	100	10	1

While the tables on the preceding pages give highs, lows, and median ranges, the appliances in your home could have values that vary greatly from those listed here. *Natural Health* magazine reported on an experiment in which they had staff members measure EMF in their offices and homes using a three-axis gaussmeter. They found background readings in their living rooms ranging from 1 to 1.2 mG. Television EMF readings were high up close to the set, from 12.5 to 24 mG. Two feet away, the readings dropped considerably—to 1.3 to 1.6 mG.

Along a wall one editor found an EMF reading of 45 mG. When he turned off the lamp that hung on that wall, the reading dropped to 12 mG. One staff member's microwave, while turned on emitted a field as strong as 120 mG up close; but four feet away, the reading dropped to 1.4 mG. Another tested his microwave, while turned off it emitted 3.7 mG up close and 1 mG four feet away. Most refrigerators were higher immediately after opening and closing. The range was 2.5 to 7.1 mG. One refrigerator, left closed, measured from 6 to 8 mG up close to the door; its back measured 25 mG.

Computers, turned off, were 1.1 to 1.3 mG. Turned on and close to the screen, readings ranged from 3.6 to 13.8 mG. But at arm's length, the reading dropped dramatically. The sides of the computers all gave off markedly higher readings than the front—as high as 62 mG up close with the computer turned on. The backs of the computers measured the highest.

Alarm clocks had literally the most alarming EMF readings, due to our habit of sleeping near them. The highest readings were 323 mG and 900 mG up close, although both dropped to 1 mG three feet away. Most electric clocks are not normally three feet away, but usually only a foot or two from our heads. Digital clocks emitted the least amount of radiation. Electric fans were also extraordinarily high. One person found a reading of 1,950 mG up close to his fan. One foot away, it dropped 65 mG, five feet away it was 2 mG. If you sit or work under a ceiling fan your exposure could be very high. How many people sleep under a ceiling fan or work in kitchens or other places under them?

Some of the differences noted above with those listed on the tables may be due to the distance from source when readings were made. The table does not list any values shorter than six inches. The measurements noted above were not as precise and so very high readings could be attributed to readings taken within an inch or two from the source.

Is Your Microwave Oven Destroying Your Health?

Rushed? No time to cook a full meal? No problem, simply pop last night's leftovers into the microwave and within minutes you have a hot steaming meal ready to eat.

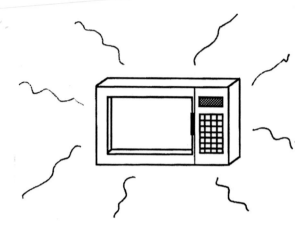

There is no question that microwave ovens have had a dramatic impact on our lives. We can cook or reheat food in a fraction of the time as it takes conventional ovens. With our busy lifestyles nowadays microwave ovens have almost become a necessity—even restaurants routinely use them. But how safe are they? And how safe is the food cooked in them?

The biggest concern about using microwave ovens is their effect on food. Anyone who has used a microwave oven knows that it can make some foods tough and rubbery. Also, cooking in microwave ovens is not uniform. We have to constantly rotate the food as it cooks to avoid overcooking in some spots and while undercooking in others. The quality and taste of food cooked in a microwave can be very different from that which comes out of conventional ovens. Is there more than taste that is different?

Unlike conventional methods of cooking, heat produced by microwave ovens is generated inside the food and not the oven itself. Radiation from nuclear bombs and other radioactive sources, likewise often creates heat and cause burns. For this reason, we often jokingly refer to "nuking" our food in the microwave. The fear many people have with microwaved food is not knowing if the molecular structure is altered during the process? Are the cells and molecules in the food possibly mutated to some unrecognizable form that can cause disease or otherwise harm our health?

That question is easy to answer—no, they aren't. Microwave ovens use high frequency radio waves, not nuclear radiation or X-rays that can cause molecular changes. These radio waves are basically the same as those used for radio broadcasting and have lower frequencies than X-rays and even visible light.

The microwaves cause certain molecules, like water, to vibrate rapidly. This creates friction which in turn produces heat. The heat in a microwave oven is derived from friction and not from the release of bonds within atoms as is done with nuclear power.

Researchers have analyzed the nutrient content of microwaved foods and have studied possible alterations that would make them different from conventionally cooked foods. There is essentially no difference. The only real health concern with microwaved food is that because it is not cooked evenly, some undercooked portions of the food may harbor living bacteria or parasites. Proper cooking, however, should eliminate this problem.

Another concern about using microwave ovens is leakage. If the microwave energy can burn food, it can burn people as well. The microwave energy inside the oven is at a much higher frequency (about 2.45 billion Hz) than the energy produced by other appliances (60 Hz). We are shielded from this energy by the casing around the inside of the oven. Leakage is a possible danger. Government standards require all microwave ovens to be built so as to prevent leakage. But as an oven ages, leaks can develop. For this reason, you might consider having a technician from the store where you purchased it or a electrical repair shop check your oven every year or two. If you have a gaussmeter you can do this yourself. Leakage, fortunately, isn't a major problem.

The biggest problem with microwave ovens comes, not from leakage of the high frequency radiation inside the oven, or from irradiated food, but from the 60 Hz electromagnetic field created by the motor and fan in the back of the unit. Just like any other appliance, microwaves emit EMFs into the environment.

The median mG of energy coming off a microwave oven is 200 at six inches, and drops to 4 at one foot. By comparison, a conventional oven has a median output of only 9 mG at six inches but 4 mG at one foot. The microwave oven emits a much stronger field up close, but a foot away the strength is about the same as a conventional oven.

A hair dryer is much worse. It emits a 300 mG field at six inches but drops to 1 mG a foot away. A vacuum cleaner also has 300 mG at six inches but only drops to 60 mG at one foot. Can openers are one of the worst. They emit a 600 mG field at six inches which drops to 150 at one foot. So microwave ovens really pose no greater health threat than any other appliance.

Can openers can emit an EMF three times as powerful as microwave ovens. In this regard your electric can opener is more dangerous than your micowave! This is especially true because, unlike the oven, you must hold on to the devise as it is being used.

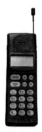

Chapter 5

ARE CELL PHONES DANGEROUS?

One of the biggest concerns regarding electromagnetic radiation is with the use of cell phones. The problem with cell phones is that when they are in use, they are up against the side of head where the full power of the electromagnetic radiation can penetrate into the brain. It wouldn't be so bad if you could speak on the phone at a distance, but cell phones are in direct contact with your face, giving your face and your brain the maximum amount of exposure to the radiation emitted by the phone.

Many experts claim that cell phones are harmless. Others disagree. Studies have been mixed. In 2008 Ronald Herberman, MD, after reviewing new data from a large international study, publicly voiced his concerns about cell phone use. Dr. Herberman comments created quit a stir because he is the director of the University of Pittsburgh Cancer Institute (UPCI), a prominent cancer research institution. He stated, "Recently I have become aware of the growing body of literature linking long-term cell phone use to possible adverse health effects including cancer. Although the evidence is still controversial, I am convinced that there are sufficient data to warrant issuing an advisory to share some precautionary advice on cell phone use.

"An international expert panel of pathologists, oncologists and public health specialists recently declared that electromagnetic fields emitted by cell phones should be considered a potential human health risk (see "The Case for Precaution in Cell Phone Use," below). To date, a number of countries including France, Germany, and India have issued recommendations that exposure to electromagnetic fields should be limited. In addition, Toronto's Department of Public Health is advising teenagers and young children to limit their use of cell phones, to avoid potential health risks.

"More definitive data that cover the health effects from prolonged cell phone use have been compiled by the World Health Organization, International Agency for Research on Cancer. However, publication has been delayed for two years. In anticipation of release of the WHO report, the attached prudent and simple precautions, intended to promote precautionary efforts to reduce exposures to cell phone electromagnetic radiation, have been reviewed by UPCI experts in neuro-oncology, epidemiology, neurosurgery and the Center for Environmental Oncology."

Studies that have been published previously have not been conclusive. Some studies show no risk. The largest published study, which appeared in the *Journal of the National Cancer Institute* in 2006, tracked 420,000 Danish cell phone users, including thousands that had used the phones for more than 10 years. It found no increased risk of cancer among those using cell phones. For these reasons the U.S. Food and Drug

Administration (FDA) states, "If there is a risk from these products—and at this point we do not know that there is—it is probably very small."

The new study is a massive project known as Interphone, involves scientists in 13 nations. It includes research on more than 5,000 cases of brain tumors. It will be another couple of years before the study is published.

Herberman says it takes too long to get answers from science and he believes people should take action now—especially when it comes to children. "Really at the heart of my concern is that we shouldn't wait for a definitive study to come out, but err on the side of being safe rather than sorry later," Herberman said.

Herberman cautions that children should use cell phones only for emergencies because their brains are still developing. Adults should keep the phone away from their heads and use the speakerphone or a wireless headset, he says. He even warns against using cell phones in public places such as a bus because it exposes others to the phone's electromagnetic fields.

The Case for Precaution in the Use of Cell Phones
(Advice from University of Pittsburgh Cancer Institute Based on Advice from an International Expert Panel)

Analysis of Recent Studies

Electromagnetic fields generated by cell phones should be considered a potential human health risk. Sufficient time has not elapsed in order for us to have conclusive data on the biological effects of cell phones and other cordless phones—a technology that is now universal.

Studies in humans do not indicate that cell phones are safe, nor do they yet clearly show that they are dangerous. But, growing evidence indicates that we should reduce exposures, while research continues on this important question.

Manufacturers report that cell and wireless phones emit electromagnetic radiation. Electromagnetic fields are likely to penetrate the brain more deeply for children than for adults. Modeling in the diagram on page 67 estimate that young children are more susceptible to electromagnetic fields due to smaller sized brains and softer brain tissue.

1) Electromagnetic fields from cell phones are estimated to penetrate the brain especially in children. (See diagram.)[1,2]

2) Living tissue is vulnerable to electromagnetic fields within the frequency bands used by cell phones (from 800 to 2200 MHz) even below the threshold of power imposed by most safety standards (1.6 W/Kg for 1g of tissue), notably an increase in the permeability of the blood-brain barrier and an increased synthesis of stress proteins.[3-6] The most recent studies, which include subjects with a history of cell phone usage for a duration of at least 10 years, show a possible association between certain benign tumors (acoustic neuromas) and some brain cancers on the side the device is used.[6-9]

However, human epidemiological studies on cell phones conducted to date cannot be conclusive. Due to their recently increased use, we are not yet able to evaluate their long term impact on health. Even where an association between exposure and cancer is well established and the risk very high — as with tobacco and lung cancer — under similar study conditions (in other words with people who smoked for less than 10 years) it would be difficult, if not impossible, to identify an increased risk of cancer, as the risk appears mostly 15 to 35 years later.[7]

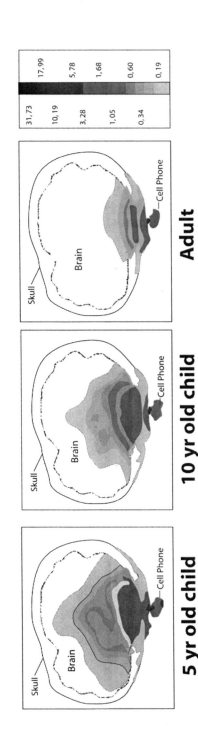

5 yr old child **10 yr old child** **Adult**

Estimation of the penetration of electromagnetic radiation from a cell phone based on age (Frequency GSM 900 Mhz) (On the right, a scale showing the *Specific Absorption Rate* at different depths, in W/kg).[1*]

---

* Researchers in the INTERPHONE study obtained comparable results with 129 more recent models cell phones (frequencies of 800 to 1800 MHz, PDC and GSM) on models of an adult brain, but have not assessed absorption in children's brains.[2]

The 10 Precautions

Given the absence of definitive proof in humans of the carcinogenic effects of electromagnetic fields of cell phones, we cannot speak about the necessity of *preventative* measures (as for tobacco or asbestos). In anticipation of more definitive data covering prolonged periods of observation, the existing data press us to share important prudent and simple measures of *precaution* for cell phone users, as have been variously suggested by several national and international reports.[6, 9, 10, 11, 12]

These measures are also likely to be important for people who are already suffering from cancer and who must avoid any external influence that may contribute to disease progression.

1. Do not allow children to use a cell phone except for emergencies. The developing organs of a fetus or child are the most likely to be sensitive to any possible effects of exposure to electromagnetic fields.

2. While communicating using your cell phone, try to keep the cell phone away from the body as much as possible. The amplitude of the electromagnetic field is one fourth the strength at a distance of two inches and fifty times lower at three feet.

Whenever possible, use the speaker-phone mode or a wireless Bluetooth headset, which has less than 1/100th of the electromagnetic emission of a normal cell phone. Use of a hands-free ear piece attachment may also reduce exposures.

3. Avoid using your cell phone in places, like a bus, where you can passively expose others to your phone's electromagnetic fields.

4. Avoid carrying your cell phone on your body at all times. Do not keep it near your body at night such as under the pillow or on a bedside table, particularly if pregnant. You can also put it on "flight" or "off-line" mode, which stops electromagnetic emissions.

5. If you must carry your cell phone on you, make sure that the keypad is positioned toward your body and the back is positioned toward the outside so that the transmitted electromagnetic fields move away from your rather than through you.

6. Only use your cell phone to establish contact or for conversations lasting a few minutes as the biological effects are directly related to the duration of exposure. For longer conversations, use a land line with a corded phone, not a cordless phone, which uses electromagnetic emitting technology similar to that of cell phones.

7. Switch sides regularly while communicating on your cell phone to spread out your exposure. Before putting your cell phone to the ear, wait until your correspondent has picked up. This limits the power of the electromagnetic field emitted near your ear and the duration of your exposure.

8. Avoid using your cell phone when the signal is weak or when moving at high speed, such as in a car or train, as this automatically increases power to a maximum as the phone repeatedly attempts to connect to a new relay antenna.

9. When possible, communicate via text messaging rather than making a call, limiting the duration of exposure and the proximity to the body.

10. Choose a device with the lowest SAR possible (SAR = Specific Absorption Rate, which is a measure of the strength of the magnetic field absorbed by the body). SAR ratings of contemporary phones by different manufacturers are available by searching for "SAR ratings cell phones" on the internet.

Conclusion

The cell phone is a remarkable invention and a breakthrough of great social importance. Our society will no longer do without cell phones. None of the members on the expert committee has stopped or intends to stop using cell telephones. This includes Dr. David Servan-Schreiber, a 16 year survivor of brain cancer. However, we, the users, must all take precautionary measures in view of recent scientific data on the biological effects of cell phone use, especially those who already have cancer.

In addition, manufacturers and service providers must also assume responsibility. It is their responsibility to provide appliances and equipment with the lowest possible risk and to constantly evolve their technology in this direction. They should also encourage consumers to use their devices in a way that is most compatible with preserving their health.

In the early 1980's, the owners of asbestos mines were reduced to bankruptcy as a result of lawsuits brought by the families of deceased exposed workers. A few years later, a key executive of Johns Manville, the most prominent company, drew lessons from the years of struggle of his industry against medical data and the scientists who were drawing attention to the risks of asbestos. He concluded with regret that greater warnings for the public, the establishment of more effective precautions, and *more extensive* medical research "could have saved lives, and probably also shareholders, the industry, and the benefits of its product."[14, 15]

We call on the cell phone companies to provide independent access to records of use so that appropriate studies can be carried out.

That is what we wish for today's cell phone industry. We do not need to ban this technology, but to adapt it – to harness it – so that it never becomes a major cause of illness.

—International Expert Committee

Bernard Asselain, MD,

Chief of the Cancer Biostatistics Service,

Curie Institute, Paris, France

Bibliography to Expert Panal Report

1. Gandhi, O.P.G. Lazzi, and C.M. Furse, *Electromagnetic Absorption in the Human Head and Neck for Cell Telephones at 835 and 1900 MHz.* IEEE Transactions on Microwave Theory and Techniques, 1996. 44(10): p. 1884-1897.

2. Cardis, E., et al., *Distribution of RF energy emitted by cell phones in anatomical structures of the brain.* Physics in Medicine and Biology, 2008. 53: p. 1-13.

3. Blank, M., *Health Risk of Electromagnetic Fields: Research on the Stress Response in The Bioinitiative Report : A Rational for a Biologically-based Public Exposure Standard for Electromagnetic Fields (ELF and RF)*. The Bioinitiative Working-Group, D. Carpenter and C. Sage, Editors. 2007

4. Johannsson, O., Evidence for effects on immune function, in *The Bioinitiative Report : A Rational for a Biologically-based Public Exposure Standard for Electromagnetic Fields (ELF and RF)*. The Bioinitiative Working-Group, D. Carpenter and C. Sage, Editors. 2007

5. Roux, D., et al., *High Frequency (900 MHz) low amplitude (5 V m-1) electromagnetic Weld: a genuine environmental stimulus that affects transcription, translation, calcium and energy charge in tomato.* Planta, 2007.

6. Commission de la sécurité des consommateurs. *AVIS RELATIF A L'INFORMATION DU CONSOMMATEUR DANS LE DOMAINE DE LA TELEPHONIE CELL 02/08.* 2008 [Cited; Available from: http://www.securiteconso.org/article647.html.

7. Walker, W.J. and B.N. Brin, *U.S. lung cancer mortality and declining cigarette tobacco consumption.* Journal of Clinical Epidemiology, 1988. 41(2): p. 179-85.

8. Hardell, L., K.H. Mild, and M. Kundi, *Evidence for brain tumors and acoustic neuromas, in The BioInitiatives Report: A Rationale for a Biologically-based Public Exposure Standard for Electromagnetic Fields (ELF and RF)*. The BioInitiative Working Group, D. Carpenter and C. Sage, Editors, 2007.

9. Board of the National Radiological Protection Board, *Cell Phones and Health*. 2004, National Radiological Protection Board: London, UK. p. 1-116.

10. Agence Française de Sécurité Sanitaire Environmentale, *Avis de l'AFSSE sur la téléphonie cell.* 2005, Agence Française de Sécurité Sanitaire Environmentale: Paris, France.

11. Ministère de la Santé. *Téléphones cells : santé et sécurité.* 2008 [cited 2008 May 16]; Available from: http://www.sante-jeunesse-sports.gouv.fr/actualite-presse/presse-sante/communiques/telephones-cells-sante-securite.html?var_recherche=portable.

12. CRIIREM Centre de Researche et d'Information Indépendantes sure les Rayonnements Electromagnétiques. *Téléphones cell: les bons réflexes!* 2006 [Cited 2008 May 26]; Available from: http://riimen.blogspirit.com/precautions protections/.

13. Sadetzki, S., et al., *Cellular phone use and risk of benign and malignant parotid gland tumors—a nationwide case-control study.* American Journal of Epidemiology, 2008. 167(4): p. 457-67.

14. Institut National de Recherche et de Sécurité, *Rayonnements électromagnétiques des téléphones portables - Mesures des émissions de divers appareils*, in *Cahiers de notes documentaires - Hygiène et sécurité du travail - N° 176.* 1999.

15. European Environment Agency, *Late Lessons from Early Warnings: the precautionary principle 1896–2000*, in *Environmental issue report.* 2001.

16. Sells, B., *What asbestos taught me about managing risk.* Harvard Business Review, 1994(March/April): p. 76-89.

Cellular Telephone Towers

Cellular telephones and towers involve radio-frequency and microwave-frequency electromagnetic fields. These are in a much higher frequency range than are the power-frequency electric and magnetic fields associated with the transmission and use of electricity.

The U.S. Federal Communications Commission (FCC) licenses communications systems that use radio-frequency and microwave electromagnetic fields and ensures that licensed facilities comply with exposure standards. Public information on this topic is published on two FCC Internet sites: http://www.fcc.gov/oet/info/ documents/bulletins/#56 and http://www.fcc.gov/oet/rfsafety/

The U.S. Food and Drug Administration also provides information about cellular telephones on its web site (http://www.fda.gov/cdrh/ocd/mobilphone.html).

Chapter 6

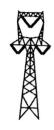

WHAT YOU CAN DO

Your EMF Environment

Scientists are still uncertain about how to best define EMF exposure. Because experiments have shown that several aspects of the fields may be relevant to biological effects. Should exposure be an average of changing magnetic field levels over some time period, or should it focus only on time spend in high fields above some threshold value? Are rapid field changes important? Does the frequency content play a role? Even though the average field level has been used widely to represent EMF exposure, it is possible that other definitions may relate more closely to any possible effects.

Another problem is that EMF in the environment is very complicated. We are usually exposed to EMF from a large number of sources every day. Fields change both in time and space. A person's EMF exposure depends to a large degree on what he or she is doing in the field at the time. For example, if you are moving and how you move within the field can increase the effects of exposure.

The best advice about reducing possible health effects from EMF exposure is to limit the amount you receive. There are a number of other ways to reduce exposures to EMFs. Some are as easy as standing back from an appliance when it is in use. Remember that magnetic fields from appliances drop off dramatically in strength with increased distance from the source.

Other EMF reduction steps, such as correcting a household wiring problem, are worth doing anyway for safety reasons. But what about more costly actions, such as burying power lines or moving out of a home? Because scientists are still debating whether EMFs are a hazard to health, it is not clear how much should be done at this time to reduce exposure. Some EMF reduction measures may create other problems. For instance, compacting power lines to reduce EMFs can increase the danger of accidental electrocution for line workers.

Does EMF Affect People with Pacemakers or Other Medical Devices?

According to the U.S. Food and Drug Administration (FDA), interference from EMF can affect various medical devices including cardiac pacemakers and implantable defibrillators. Most current research in this area focuses on higher frequency sources such as cellular phones, citizens band radios, wireless computer links, microwave signals, radio and television transmitters, and paging transmitters.

Sources such as welding equipment, power lines at electric generating plants, and rail transportation equipment can produce lower frequency EMF strong enough to interfere with some models of pacemakers and defibrillators. The occupational exposure guidelines developed by ACGIH state that workers with cardiac pacemakers should not be exposed to a 60-Hz magnetic field greater than 1 gauss (1,000 mG) or a 60-Hz electric field greater than 1 kilovolt per meter (1,000 V/m). Workers who are concerned about EMF exposure effects on pacemakers, implantable defibrillators, or other implanted electronic medical devices should consult their doctors or industrial hygienists.

Nonelectronic metallic medical implants (such as artificial joints, pins, nails, screws, and plates) can be affected by high magnetic fields such as those from magnetic resonance imaging (MRI) devices and aluminum refining equipment, but are generally unaffected by the lower fields from most other sources.

The FDA MedWatch program is collecting information about medical device problems thought to be associated with exposure to or interference from EMF.

Anyone experiencing a problem that might be due to such interference is encouraged to call and report it (800-332-1088).

EMF Measurements

The EMFs in and around your home can be determined using a gaussmeter. A gaussmeter is a handheld device that measures magnetic field strength. There are two basic types. Three-axis meters, which measure the three directional components of a magnetic field, these cost hundreds of dollars each. Single-axis meters cost less but measure in only one direction, and therefore, take some work to get an accurate reading. For the average person, a single-axis meter is sufficient. Prices for adequate ones start at around $150. Gaussmeters are advertised in most of the EMF periodicals listed in the appendix.

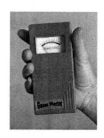 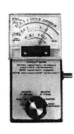 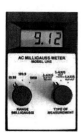

Handheld gaussmeters

Elevated EMFs within a home are often caused by errors made in the electrical wring either during construction of the house, or during modifications made later. These minor violations of the National Electrical Code are often undetected because they do not affect the performance of the electrical system. But they can create substantially elevated EMFs. Examples of this are tying neutrals together in a junction box, incorrect bonding of the neutral or ground to the plumbing, or use of an incorrect cable in multi-way switches. Situations such as these often create large areas within the home of very high elevated fields. These problems can be tracked down and corrected by bringing the wiring into compliance with the Electrical Code.

Because people are becoming aware of the possible hazards of EMFs, companies have recently emerged that can come to your home and measure EMFs for you. These independent measurement technicians will conduct EMF measurements for a fee, usually around $100-$200. They can measure external EMF that may affect you as well as sources in your home, particularly hidden ones such as wiring behind walls or under floors. Basically an EMF survey will pinpoint areas of elevated radiation in the home. The advantage of this is that once you know where the "hot spots" are in your home you can get them corrected by modifying the wiring or take steps to avoid prolonged proximity to them. In some cities, these companies are listed in the yellow pages of the telephone book under the heading "Engineers, environmental."

You may not need to buy a gaussmeter or hire an independent technician to measure your home for EMFs. For specific information about EMFs from a particular power line, contact the utility that operates the line. Most utilities will conduct EMF measurements for customers at no charge. If you can get your home measured by a utility company you may not need to bother getting a meter. Although, if you have a meter of your own or hire someone to do it, you can usually get more detailed measurements from around the home and near appliances.

The graph on the following page shows how one magnetic field measured every 24 seconds over a 24-hour period appeared. Field exposure at home may be low. The occasional spikes (short exposures to high field) occurred when the person drove or walked under or over power lines or was close to appliances in the home or office.

Some studies have used these automatic gaussmeters to measure human exposure to magnetic fields. These studies tend to show that appliances and building wiring contribute to the

Example of 24-Hour Magnetic Field Exposure

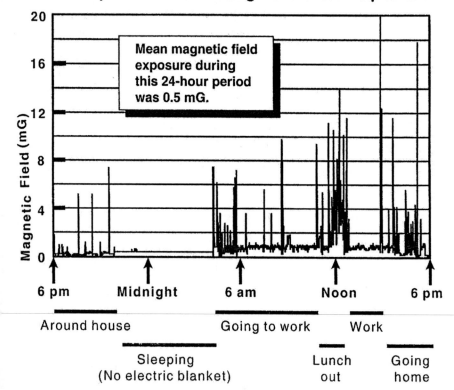

Mean magnetic field exposure during this 24-hour period was 0.5 mG.

Random sample of the magnetic field exposure over a 24-hour period. The test subject works in an office with a computer and lives in an area with relatively low background EMF.

low-level background magnetic field exposure that most people receive. People living close to large power lines tend to have higher overall field exposures. However, as shown here, there can be much individual variation among homes.

What About Products Advertised As Producing Low or Reduced Magnetic Fields?

Virtually all electrical appliances and devices emit electric and magnetic fields. The strengths of the fields vary appreciably both between types of devices and among manufacturers and models of the same type of device. Some appliance manufacturers are designing new models that, in general, have lower EMF than older models. As a result, the words "low field" or "reduced field" may be relative to older models and not necessarily relative to other manufacturers or devices. At this time, there are no domestic or international standards or guidelines limiting the EMF emissions of appliances.

The U.S. government has set no standards for magnetic fields from computer monitors or video display terminals (VDTs). The Swedish Confederation of Professional Employees (TCO) established in 1992 a standard recommending strict limits on the EMF emissions of computer monitors. The VDTs should produce magnetic fields of no more than 2 mG at a distance of 30 cm (about 1 ft) from the front surface of the monitor and 50 cm (about 1 ft 8 in) from the sides and back of the monitor. The TCO'92 standard has become a *de facto* standard in the VDT industry worldwide. A 1999 standard, promulgated by the Swedish TCO (known as the TCO'99 standard), provides for international and environmental labeling of personal computers. Many computer monitors marketed in the U.S. are certified as compliant with TCO'99 and are thereby assured to produce low magnetic fields.

Beware of advertisements claiming that the federal government has certified that the advertised equipment produces little or no EMF. The federal government has no such general certification program for the emissions of low-frequency EMF. The U.S. Food and Drug Administration's Center for Devices and Radiological Health (CDRH) does certify medical equipment and equipment producing high levels of ionizing radiation or microwave radiation. Information about certain devices as well as general information about EMF is available from the CDRH at 888-463-6332.

Reducing Your Exposure

Do you remember as a kid sitting close to the television and having your mother say to you, "Don't sit so close to the screen, it will ruin your eyes?" Perhaps you have used these same words on your own kids. The fact that televisions and other electrical devices emit radiation seems to be obvious. We have suspected it since the first television sets were made and long before knowledge of EMF dangers were widely known. The first thing you can do to reduce your exposure to EMFs is to move farther away from appliances, especially while they are in operation. Since radiation drops rather quickly, this is the easiest thing you can do to protect yourself.

For a television, sit as far back from the screen as possible. Getting a larger screen so you can see better from a distance isn't necessarily a good solution because a larger screen will emit more radiation. The new LCD flat panel TVs emit less radiation than the old picture tube sets.

Computers have become a common tool around the office and the home. Many of us spend hours every day staring into the screen of a computer. Most people work far to close to

84

their screens. Sit at arm's length from the screen and check the distance from other appliances. If you spend extended periods of time in front of a computer monitor, you should consider some of the newer lower radiation monitors. Those monitors, which are labeled "low radiation", comply with the MPRII standard set by the Swedish government which requires low levels of EMF.

Many appliances such a electric razors and hair dryers produce very high EMFs up close, but since they are used for only a short period of time it is generally believed that their effects are of minor concern. The greatest threat is from appliances that we use up close for long periods of time—sitting under a lamp, sleeping next to a clock, or working under a ceiling fan, for example.

Alarm clocks, especially the older, dial-face models are notorious EMF-emitters. Push your clock a few feet away from the pillow.

Simple Steps to Reduce EMF

Simple precautionary steps such as the following, can be the most effective way to reduce most EMF exposure:

- Increase the distance between yourself and the EMF source—sit at arm's length from your computer terminal.
- Avoid unnecessary proximity to high EMF sources—don't let children play directly under power lines or on top of power transformers for underground lines.
- Reduce time spent within a field—turn off your computer monitor and other electrical appliances when you aren't using them.

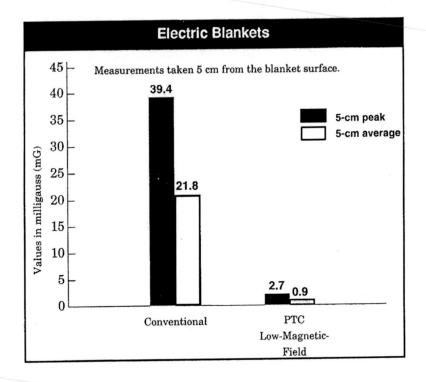

Electric Blankets

Measurements taken 5 cm from the blanket surface.

Values in milligauss (mG)

- 5-cm peak
- 5-cm average

Conventional: 39.4, 21.8

PTC Low-Magnetic-Field: 2.7, 0.9

Some of the worst appliances are those that are used against the body like electric blankets, heating pads, and heated water beds. These devices have shown to have adverse effects on reproductive and children's health. Not using electric blankets or use them only to heat the bed and then unplugging them prior to use would eliminate harmful exposure. Another option available is using low-field electric blankets that have just come on the market.

As noted earlier, cellular phones have emerged as a possible troublemaker because they are used a close distances. Some people spend many hours every day on them. The portable models, which contain the power supply and antenna in the handset, are of greatest concern; car phones are less worrisome.

Also check the position of appliances in your home. Electrical equipment stacked against the wall can radiate EMF through the wall into the adjoining rooms. Remember electromagnetic energy is not blocked by walls. The EMFs emitted from behind electrical appliances are often much stronger than those released out the front. Emissions can be as strong as 50 mG or more on the other side of a wall where an appliance sits.

If you have a television against the wall you definitely do not want to have your child sleeping in a crib on the other side. This has been suggested as a possible cause for sudden infant death syndrome. Check the position of computers, TVs, the refrigerator, microwave, and other appliances. It is best to have their backs turned toward the outside wall so EMFs emitted from the rear of appliances goes out the home rather than into another room where they could affect people.

With the aid of a gaussmeter or environmental engineer you can discover the hidden "hot spots" in your home such as behind walls or under the floor. Once you know where the hot spots are, you can move things around accordingly. If you discover the wall behind your pillow measures 10 mG, for example, move the bed to the opposite wall, or change rooms. You often find a hot spot on the other side of the wall where the electrical power comes into the house. Wall sockets and outlets are hot spots where wiring comes together near the surface of wall. You should avoid sleeping or sitting too close to these. The biggest problem is wiring inside the wall where you can't see it. This is were a gaussmeter is really handy to have as it can detect where the wiring is and the strength of the field.

Louis Slesin, editor of *Microwave News*, which reports on EMF health effects, suggests, whenever possible, reducing exposure to less than 1 milligauss. Many home appliances, for instance, emit extremely high levels of EMFs—often over 100 mG—when you are up close to them. Fortunately, the field usually falls off relatively quickly over a short distance, usually within a few feet.

The U.S. Environmental protection Agency, provides a toll-free public information telephone line to answer EMF-related questions and direct callers to further sources of information.

The EMF "Infoline" number is 1-800-363-2383.

(In Washington D.C., call 484-1803)

Microwave News, a bimonthly newsletter, covers EMF health effects. If you would like a list of companies that sell gaussmeters, or a list of low EMF computers, send your request with a self-addressed, stamped, business-sized envelope, plus $1 to:

Microwave News, P.O. Box 1799, Grand Central Station, New York, NY 10163 or visit their website at www.microwavenews.com.

Appendix

REFERENCES AND RESOURCES

EMF Periodicals

Between the Lines, Center for Energy Information, Augusta, Maine. Call 800-947-8765.

EMF Health & Safety Digest, Minneapolis, Call 612-623-4600.

EMF Health Report, Information ventures, Inc., Philadelphia. Call 215-732-9083

EMF News, Washington, D.C. Call 202-508-5425.

Microwave News, New York. Call 212-517-2800. Will provide a current list of gaussmeter manufacturers. Send $1.00 to Microwave News, P.O. Box 1799, Grand Central Station, New York, NY 10163.

Articles and Books About the EMF Controversy

Brodeur, P. 1993. *The Great Power-Line Cover-Up*. Little, Brown, New York.

"EcoCancers: Do Environmental Factors Underlie a Breast Cancer Epidemic?" pp. 10-13 in *Science News*, July 3, 1993.

"Electromagnetic Fields," pp. 354-359 in *Consumer Reports*, May 1994.

"EMFs Run Aground," pp. 124-127 in *Science News*, August 21, 1993.

"Findings Point to Complexity of Health Effects of Electric, Magnet Fields," pp. 27-33 in *Chemical and Engineering News*, July 1994.

Taubes, G. "Fields of Fear," pp. 94-108 in *Atlantic Monthly*, November 1994.

References

These references are grouped by the major topics covered in this publication. Most should be available in technical libraries. Check your local universities or medical schools.

Basic Science

Paris, D.T., and F.K. Hurd. 1969. *Basic Electromagnetic Theory*, McGraw Hill.

Kovetz A. *Electromagnetic Theory.* New York: Oxford University Press (2000).

Vanderlinde J. *Classical Electromagnetic Theory.* New York: Wiley (1993).

EMF Levels and Exposures

Bowman, J.D., et al. 1992. *Electric and Magnetic Field Exposure, Chemical Exposure, and Leukemia Risk in "Electrical" Occupations.* Prepared by the University of Southern California for the Electric Power Research Institute, Palo Alto, Calif.

Bracken, T.D., and R.F. Rankin (Principal Investigators). 1994. *EMDEX Project Residential Study Final Report.* Prepared by T. Dan Bracken, Inc., for the Electric Power Research Institute, Palo Alto, Calif.

Gauger, J.r. 1985. "Household Appliance Magnetic Field Survey," *IEEE Transactions on Power Apparatus and Systems PAS* 104 (9): 2436-2444.

Stearns, R.D., M.W. Tuominen, and V.L. Chartier. 1992. "Magnetic Field Characterization for the Bonneville Power Administration's 500-, 230-, and 115-kV Transmission Line Systems." Abstract P-26. *The Annual Review of Research on Biological Effects of Electric and Magnetic Fields from the Generation, Delivery, and Use of Electricity.* W/L Associates, Ltd., Frederick, Md.

Zaffanella, L.E., (Principal Investigator). 1993. *Survey of Residential Magnetic Field Sources.* Final Report TR-102759

(2 volumes). Prepared by the High Voltage Transmission Research Center for the Electric Power Research Institute, Palo Alto, Calif.

EMF Measurement Protocols

IEEE Magnetic Field Task Force of the AC Fields Working Group of the Corona Field Effects Subcommittee of the Transmission and Distribution Committee, "A Protocol for Spot Measurements fo Residential Power Frequency Magnetic Fields," *IEEE Transactiosn on Power Delivery 1993*, July, 8 (3): 1386-94.

National EMF Measurement Protocol Group. 1994. *Power Frequency Magnetic Fields: A Protocol for Conducting Spot Measurements in Residential Settings*.

Yost, M.G., G.M. Lee, D. Duane, J. Fisch, and R.R. Neutra. 1992. "California Protocol for Measuring 60 Hz Magnetic Fields in Residences," *Applied Occupational Environmental Hygiene*, November, 7(11): 772-77.

EMF Standards and Regulations

ACGIH (American Conference of Governmental Industrial Hygienists). 1994. 1994-1995 *Threshold Limit Values for Chemical Substances and Physical Agents and Biological Exposure Indices*. Cincinnati. ISBN 1-882417-06-2.

Electro-Magnetic Health Effects Committee. 1992. "Regulatory Issues," Chap. 6 in *Health Effects of Exposure to Powerline-Frequency Electric and Magnetic Fields*. Public Utility Commission of Texas, Austin, Tex.

IRPA/INIRC (International Nonionizing Radiation Committee of the International Radiation Protection Association). 1990. "Interim Guidelines on Limits of Exposure to 50/60-Hz Electric and Magnetic Fields, *Health Physics* 58: 113-122.

Maddock, B.J. 1992. "Exposure Limits Around the World," *Electric and Magnetic Fields in the Workplace Proceedings*, October 21-23, Paris. International Commission on Occupational Health Radiation and Work Committee.

SWEDAC (Swedish Board for Technical Assistance). 1990. *User's Handbook for Evaluating Visual Display Units*. MPR 1990:10 1990-12-31. SWEDAC, Bords, Sweden.

TCO (Tjanstemannens Central Organisation, Swedish Confederation of Professional Employees). 1994. *Screen Facts*. Stockholm, TCO Information Center, Chicago.

Residential Childhood Cancer Studies
(The following references are in chronological order.)

Wertheimer, N., and E. Leeper. 1979. "Electrical Wiring Configurations and Childhood Cancer," *American Journal of Epidemiology* 109: 273-284.

Fulton, J.P., S. Cobb, L. Preble, L. Leone, and E. Forman. 1980. "Electrical Wiring Configurations and Childhood Leukemia in Rhode Island," *American Journal of Epidemiology* 111: 292-296.

Tomenius, L. 1986. "50-Hz Electromagnetic Environment and the Incidence of Childhood Tumors in Stockholm County," *Bioelectromagnetics* 7: 191-207.

Savitz, D.A., H. Wachtel, F.A. Barnes, E.M. John, and J.G. Tvrdik. 1988. "Case-Contorl Study of Childhood Cancer and Exposure to 60-Hz Magnetic Fields," *American Journal of Epidemiology* 128: 21-38.

Coleman, M.P., C.M.J. Bell, H.L. Taylor, and M.P. Zakelj. 1989. "Leukaemia and Residence Near Electricity Transmission Equipment: A Case-Control Study," *British Journal of Cancer* 60: 793-798.

Myers, A., A.D. Clayden, R.A. Cartwright, and S.C. Cartwright. 1990. "Childhood Cancer and Overhead Powerlines: A Case-Control Study," *British Journal of Cancer* 62: 1008-1014.

London, S., D.C. Thomas, J.D. Gowman, E. Sobel, T.C. Cheng, and J.M. Peters. 1991. "Exposure to Residential Electric and Magnetic Fields and Risk of Childhood Leukemia," *American Journal of Epidemiology* 134: 923-937.

Lowenthal, R.M., J.B. Panton, M.J. Baikie, and J. N. Lickiss. 1991. "Exposure to Hight Tension Power Lines and Childhood Leukaemia: A Pilot Study," *Medical Journal of Australia* 155: 347.

Feychting, M., and A. Ahlbom. 1993. "Magnetic Fields and Cancer in Children Residing near Swedish High-Voltage Power Lines," *American Journal of Epidemiology* 138: 467-481.

Olsen, J.H., A. Nielsen, and G. Schulgen. 1993. "Residence near High Voltage Facilities and the Risk of Cancer in Children," *British Medical Journal* 307: 891-895.

Verkasalo, P.K., et al. 1993. "Risk of Cancer in Finnish Children Living Close to Power Lines," *British Medical Journal* 307: 895-899.

Petridou, E., et al. 1993. "Age of Exposure to Infections and Risk of Childhood Leukaemia," *British Medical Journal* 307: 774.

Fajardo-Gutierrez, A., et al. 1993. "Close Residence to High Electric Voltage Lines and Its Association with Children with Leukemia" (In Spanish), *Boletin Medico del Hospital Infantil de Mexico* 50: 32-38.

Ahlbom, A., Feychting, M. Koskenvuo, J.H. Olsen, E. Pukkala, G. Schulgen, and P. Verkasalo. 1993. "Electromagnetic Fields and Childhood Cancer," *Lancet* 342: 1295-1296.

Residential Adult Cancer Studies

(The following references are in chronological order.)

Wertheimer, N., and E. Leeper. 1982. "Adult Cancer Related to Electrical Wires near the Home," *International Journal of Epidemiology* 11: 345-355.

McDowell, M.E. 1986. "Mortality of Persons Resident in the Vicinity of Electricity Transmission Facilities," *British Journal of Cancer* 53: 271-279.

Severson, R.K., R.G. Stevens, W.T. Kaune, D.B. Thomas, L. Heuser, S. Davis, and L.E. Sever. 1988. "Acute Nonlymphoctic Leukemia and Residential Exposure to Power Frequency Magnetic Fields," *American Journal of Epidemiology* 128: 10-20.

Coleman, M.P., C.M.J. Bell, H.L. Taylor, and M.P. Zakelj. 1989. "Leukaemia and Residence near Electricity Transmission Equipment: A Case-Control Study," *British Journal of Cancer* 60: 793-798.

Youngson, J.H.A.M., A.D. Clayden, A. Myers, and R.A. Cartwright. 1991. "A Case-Control Study of Adult Hematological Malignancies in Relation to Overhead Powerlines," *British Journal of Cancer* 63: 977-985.

Eriksson, M., and M. Karisson. 1992. "Occupational and Other Environmental Factors and Multiple Myeloma: A Population Based Case-Control Study," *British Journal of Industrial Medicine* 49: 95-103.

Feychting, M., A. Ahlbom. 1992. *Magnetic Fields and Cancer in People Residing Near Swedish High Voltage Power Lines*, Institute of Environmental Medicine, Karolinska Institute, Stockholm.

Schreiber, G.H., G.M.H. Swaen, J.M.M. Meijers, J.J.M. Slangen, and F. Sturmans. 1993. "Cancer Mortality and Residence Near Electricity Transmission Eequipment: A Retrospective Cohort Study," *International Journal of Epidemiology* 22: 9-15.

Cancer Clusters

Anonymous. 1990. "State Health Studies in Connecticut and North Carolina Refute Brodeur's 'Cancer Clusters,'" *Transmission/Distribution Health & Safety Report* 8: 6, 9-10.

Neutra, R.R., and E. Glazer. 1993. *An Evaluation of an Alleged Cancer Cluster Among Teachers at the Stater School Between 1973 and 1992*. California Department of Health Services, Berkeley, Calif.

(Several papers on the clustering of health events can also be found in the *American Journal of Epidemiology*, Vol. 132: Supplement, June 1990.)

Occupational EMF Cancer Studies

Coogan PF, Clapp RW, Newcomb PA, Wenzl TB, Bogdan G, Mittendorf R, Baron JA & Longnecker MP. Occupational exposure to 60-Hertz magnetic fields and risk of breast cancer in women. *Epidemiology* 7:459-464 (1996).

Floderus B, Persson T, Stenlund C, Wennberg A, Ost A, & Knave B. Occupational exposure to electromagnetic fields in relation to leukemia and brain tumors: a case-control study in Sweden. *Cancer Causes Control* 4:465-476 (1993).

Floderus B, Tornqvist S, & Stenlund C. Incidence of selected cancers in Swedish railway workers, 1961-79. *Cancer Causes Control* 5:189-194 (1994).

Sorahan T, Nichols L, van Tongeren M, & Harrington JM. Occupational exposure to magnetic fields relative to mortality from brain tumours: updated and revised findings from a study of United Kingdom electricity generation and transmission workers, 1973–97. *Occupational and Environmental Medicine* 58(10):626-630 (2001).

Johansen C, & Olsen JH Risk of cancer among Danish utility workers - A nationwide cohort study. *American Journal of Epidemiology*, 147:548-555 (1998).

Kheifets LI, Gilbert ES, Sussman SS, Guenel P, Sahl JD, Savitz DA, & Theriault G. Comparative analyses of the studies of magnetic fields and cancer in electric utility workers: studies from France, Canada, and the United States. *Occupational and Environmental Medicine* 56(8):567-574 (1999).

London SJ, Bowman JD, Sobel E, Thomas DC, Garabrant DH, Pearce N, Bernstein L & Peters JM . Exposure to magnetic fields among electrical workers in relation to leukemia risk in Los Angeles County. *American Journal of Industrial Medicine* 26:47-60 (1994).

Matanoski GM, Breysse PN & Elliott EA. Electromagnetic field exposure and male breast cancer. *Lancet* 337:737 (1991).

Sahl JD, Kelsh MA, & Greenland S. Cohort and nested case-control studies of hematopoietic cancers and brain cancer among utility worker. *Epidemiology* 4:21-32 (1994).

Savitz DA & Loomis DP. Magnetic field exposure in relation to leukemia and brain cancer mortality among electric utility workers. *American Journal of Epidemiology* 141:123-134(1995).

Sorahan T, Nichols L, van Tongeren M, & Harrington JM. Occupational exposure to magnetic fields relative to mortality from brain tumours: updated and revised findings from a study of United Kingdom electricity generation and transmission workers, 1973–97. *Occupational and Environmental Medicine* 58:626-630 (2001).

Thériault G, Goldberg M, Miller AB, Armstrong B, Guénel P, Deadman J, Imbernon E, To T, Chevalier A, Cyr D, & Wall C. Cancer risks associated with occupational exposure to magnetic fields among electric utility workers in Ontario and Quebec, Canada and France: 1970–1989. *American Journal of Epidemiology* 139:550-572 (1994).

Tynes T, Jynge H, & Vistnes AI. Leukemia and brain tumors in Norwegian railway workers, a nested case-control study. *American Journal of Epidemiology* 139:645-653 (1994).

Some National Reviews of EMF Research

Advisory Group on Non-Ionizing Radiation. 1992. *Electromagnetic Fields and Cancer* 3(1). National Radiological Protection Board. Chilton, Didcot, Oxon, U.K.

Expert Group of the Danish ministry of Health on Non-Ionizing Radiation. 1993. *Report on the Risk of Cancer in Children with Homes Exposed to 50 Hz Magnetic Fields from High-Voltage Installations.* Danish Ministry of Health, Copenhagen.

Guenel, P., and J. Lellouch. 1993. *Synthesis of the Literature on Health Effects from Very Low Frequency Electric and Magnetic Fields.* INSERM, National Institute of Health and Medical Research, Paris.

Oak Ridge Associated Universities Panel. 1992. *Health Effects of Low-Frequency Electric and Magnetic Fields.* ORAU 92/F8. prepared for the Committee on Interagency Radiation Research and Policy Coordination. U.S. Government Printing Office: GPO #029-000-00443-9.

Peach, H.G., W.J. Bonwick, R. Scanlan, and T. Wyse. 1992. *Report of the Panel on Electromagnetic Fields and Health to the Victorian Government.* Minister of Health, Melbourne, Australia.

Science Advisory Board. 1992. *Potential Carcinogenicity of Electric and Magnetic Fields*. EPA SAB-RAC-92-013. U.S. Evnironmental Protection Agency, Washington, D.C.

Swedish National Board for Electrical Safety. 1993. *Revised Assessment of Magnetic Fields and Health Hazards*. Stockholm.

Electricity Use and Cancer Rates

Jackson, J.D. 1992. "Are the Stray 60-Hz Electromagnetic Fields Associated with the Distribution and Use of Electric Power a Significant Cause of Cancer?" *Proceedings of the National Academy of Sciences* 89: 3508-3510.

Kujawa, L.J., et al. 1992. *Electric Power Trends 1992*. Arthur Anderson & Co., Atlanta, and Cambridge Energy Research Associates, Inc., Cambridge, Mass.

Miller, B.A., et al., eds. 1992. *Cancer Statistics Review: 1973-1989*. NIH Pub. No. 92-2789. National Cancer Institute, Bethesda, Md.

Savitz, D.A. 1993. "Health Effects of Low-Frequency Electric and Magnetic Fields," *Environmental Science and Technology* 27: 52-54.

Some Noncancer EMF Studies of Humans

Brent, R.L., W.E. Gordon, W.R. Bennett, and D.A. Beckman. 1993. "Reproductive and Teratologic Effects of Electromagnetic Fields," *Reproductive Toxicology* 7: 535-580.

Juutilainen, J., P. Matilainen, S. Saarikoski, E. Laara, and S. Suonio. 1993. "Early Pregnancy Loss and Exposure to 50-Hz Magnetic Fields," *Bioelectromagnetics* 14: 229-236.

Lindbohm, M.L., et al. 1992. "Magnetic Fields of Video Display Terminals and Spontaneous Abortion," *American Journal of Epidemiology* 136: 1041-1051.

McMahan s. J. Ericson, and J. Meyer. 1994. "Depressive Symptomatology in Women and Residential Proximity to High-Voltage Transmission Lines," *American Journal of Epidemiology* 139: 58-63.

Poole, C., et al. 1993. "Depressive Symptoms and Headaches in Relation to Proximity to an Alternating-Current Transmission Line Right-of-Way," *American Journal of Epidemiology* 137: 318-330.

Rea, W.J., et al. 1991. "Electromagnetic Field Sensitivity," *Journal of Bioelectricity* 10: 241-256.

Roman, E., V. Beral, M. Pelerin, and C. Hermon. 1992. "Spontaneous Abortion and Work with VisualDisplay Units," *British Journal of Industrial Medicine* 49: 507-512.

Laboratory Animal EMF Studies

Anderson LE, Boorman GA, Morris JE, Sasser LB, Mann PC, Grumbein SL, Hailey JR, McNally A, Sills RC & Haseman JK. Effect of 13-week magnetic field exposures on DMBA-initiated mammary gland carcinomas in female Sprague-Dawley rats. *Carcinogenesis* 20:1615-1620 (1999).

Baum A, Mevissen M, Kamino K, Mohr U & Löscher W. A histopathological study on alterations in DMBA-induced mammary carcinogenesis in rats with 50 Hz, 100 mT magnetic field exposure. *Carcinogenesis* 16:119-125 (1995).

Babbitt JT, Kharazi AI, Taylor JMG, Rafferty CN, Kovatch R, Bonds CB, Mirell SG, Frumkin E, Dietrich F, Zhuang D & Hahn TJM. Leukemia/lymphoma in mice exposed to 60-Hz magnetic fields: Results of the chronic exposure study TR-110338. Los Angeles: Electric Power Research Institute (EPRI) (1998).

Babbitt JT, Kharazi AI, Taylor JMG, Rafferty CN, Kovatch R, Bonds CB, Mirell SG, Frumkin E, Dietrich F, Zhuang D & Hahn TJM. Leukemia/lymphoma in mice exposed to 60-Hz magnetic fields: Results of the chronic exposure study, Second Edition. Electric Power Research Institute (EPRI) and B. C. Hydro, Palo Alto, California and Burnaby, British Columbia, Canada (1999).

Boorman GA, Anderson LE, Morris JE, Sasser LB, Mann PC, Grumbein SL, Hailey JR, McNally A, Sills RC & Haseman JK. Effect of 26-week magnetic field exposures in a DMBA initiation-promotion mammary gland model in Sprague-Dawley rats. *Carcinogenesis* 20:899-904 (1999).

Boorman GA, McCormick DL, Findlay JC, Hailey JR, Gauger JR, Johnson TR, Kovatch RM, Sills RC & Haseman JK. Chronic toxicity/oncogenicity of 60 Hz (power frequency) magnetic fields in F344/N rats. *Toxicological Pathology* 27:267-278 (1999).

Boorman GA, McCormick DL, Ward JM, Haseman JK & Sills RC. Magnetic fields and mammary cancer in rodents: A critical review and evaluation of published literature. *Radiation Research* 153:617-626 (2000).

Boorman GA, Rafferty CN, Ward JM & Sills RC. Leukemia and lymphoma incidence in rodents exposed to low-frequency magnetic fields. *Radiation Research* 153:627-636 (2000).

Ekström T, Mild KH & Holmberg B. Mammary tumours in Sprague-Dawley rats after initiation with DMBA followed by exposure to 50 Hz electromagnetic fields in a promotional scheme. *Cancer Letters* 123:107-111 (1998).

Mandeville R, Franco E, Sidrac-Ghali S, Paris-Nadon L, Rocheleau N, Mercier G, Desy M & Gaboury L. Evaluation of the potential carcinogenicity of 60 Hz linear sinusoidal continuous-wave magnetic fields in Fisher F344 rats. *Federation of the American Society of Experimental Biology Journal* 11:1127-1136 (1997).

McCormick DL, Boorman GA, Findlay JC, Hailey JR, Johnson TR, Gauger JR, Pletcher JM, Sills RC & Haseman JK. Chronic toxicity/oncogenicity of 60 Hz (power frequency) magnetic fields in B6C3F1 mice. *Toxicological Pathology* 27:279-285 (1999).

Mevissen M, Lerchl A, Szamel M & Löscher W. Exposure of DMBA-treated female rats in a 50Hz, 50 microTesla magnetic field: Effects on mammary tumor growth, melatonin levels and T-lymphocyte activation. *Carcinogenesis* 17:903-910 (1996).

Yasui M, Kikuchi T, Ogawa M, Otaka Y, Tsuchitani M & Iwata H. Carcinogenicity test of 50 Hz sinusoidal magnetic fields in rats. *Bioelectromagnetics* 18:531-540 (1997).

Laboratory Cellular EMF Studies

Balcer-Kubiczek EK, Harrison GH, Zhang XF, Shi ZM, Abraham JM, McCready WA, Ampey LL, III, Meltzer SJ, Jacobs MC, & Davis CC. Rodent cell transformation and immediate early gene expression following 60-Hz magnetic field exposure. *Environmental Health Perspectives* 104:1188-1198 (1996).

Boorman GA, Owen RD, Lotz WG & Galvin MJ, Jr. Evaluation of *in vitro* effects of 50 and 60 Hz magnetic fields in regional EMF exposure facilities. *Radiation Research* 153:648-657 (2000).

Lacy-Hulbert A, Metcalfe JC, & Hesketh R. Biological responses to electromagnetic fields. *Federation of the American Society of Experimental Biology (FASEB) Journal* 12:395-420 (1998).

Morehouse CA & Owen RD. Exposure of Daudi cells to low-frequency magnetic fields does not elevate MYC steady-state mRNA levels. *Radiation Research* 153:663-669 (2000).

Snawder JE, Edwards RM, Conover DL & Lotz WG. Effect of magnetic field exposure on anchorage-independent growth of a promoter-sensitive mouse epidermal cell line (JB6). *Environmental Health Perspectives* 107:195-198 (1999).

Wey HE, Conover DL, Mathias P, Toraason MA & Lotz WG. 50-Hz magnetic field and calcium transients in Jurkat cells: Results of a research and public information dissemination (RAPID) program study. *Environmental Health Perspectives* 108:135-140 (2000).

Studies of Melatonin and EMF

Lee, J.M., et al. 1993. "Melatonin Secretion and Puberty in Femal Lambs Exposed to Environmental Electric and Magnetic Fields," *Biology of Reproduction* 49: 857-864.

Liburdy, R.P., T.R. Sloma, R. Sokolic, and P. Yaswen. 1993. "ELF Magnetic Fields, Breast Cancer, and Melatonin: 60 Hz Fields Block Melatonin's Oncostatic Action on ER Breast Cancer Cell Proliferation," *Journal of Pineal Research* 14: 89-97.

Reiter, R.J. 1992. "Alterations of the Circadian Melatonin Rhythm by the Electromagnetic Spectrum: A Study in Environmental Toxicology," *Regulatory Toxicology and Pharmacology* 15: 226-244.

Wilson, B.W., R.G. Stevens, and L.E. Anderson. 1989. "Minireview: Neuroendocrine Mediated Effects of Electromagnetic Field Exposure: Possible Role of the Pineal Gland," *Life Sciences* 45: 1319-1332.

INDEX

Made in the USA